Hot Mamas

Hot Mamas

The Ultimate Guide to Staying Sexy Throughout Your Pregnancy and the Months Beyond

LOU PAGET

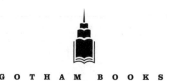

GOTHAM BOOKS

GOTHAM BOOKS

Published by Penguin Group (USA) Inc.
37 Hudson Street, New York, New York 10014, U.S.A.

Penguin Group (Canada), 10 Alcorn Avenue, Toronto, Ontario, Canada M4V 3B2 (a division of Pearson Penguin Canada Inc.); Penguin Books Ltd, 80 Strand, London WC2R 0RL, England; Penguin Ireland, 25 St Stephen's Green, Dublin 2, Ireland (a division of Penguin Books Ltd); Penguin Group (Australia), 250 Camberwell Road, Camberwell, Victoria 3124, Australia (a division of Pearson Australia Group Pty Ltd); Penguin Books India Pvt Ltd, 11 Community Centre, Panchsheel Park, New Delhi – 110 017, India; Penguin Group (NZ), Cnr Airborne and Rosedale Roads, Albany, Auckland, New Zealand (a division of Pearson New Zealand Ltd); Penguin Books (South Africa) (Pty) Ltd, 24 Sturdee Avenue, Rosebank, Johannesburg 2196, South Africa

Penguin Books Ltd, Registered Offices: 80 Strand, London WC2R 0RL, England

Published by Gotham Books, a division of Penguin Group (USA) Inc.

First printing, January 2005
1 3 5 7 9 10 8 6 4 2

Copyright © 2005 by Lou Paget
All rights reserved

Grateful acknowledgment is made for permission to reprint the following:

An excerpt from *Sex Toys 101* by Rachel Venning and Claire Cavanah,
copyright © 2003 by Rachel Venning and Claire Cavanah. Reprinted with
the permission of Simon & Schuster Adult Publishing Group.

Three images from *Body Talk: An A–Z Guide to Women's Health*
by Dr. Jules Black, copyright © 1988 by Dr. Jules Black.
Reprinted by permission from the author.

Ten illustrations by Robert Dunlap, copyright © Robert Dunlap.
Reprinted by permission of Robert Dunlap, RED Productions, Inc.

Images from the *Liberator Bedroom Adventure Gear* Catalogue. Reprinted by
permission of Don Cohen, President, Liberator Shapes/OneUp Innovations.

Gotham Books and the skyscraper logo are trademarks of Penguin Group (USA) Inc.

LIBRARY OF CONGRESS CATALOGING-IN-PUBLICATION DATA
HAS BEEN APPLIED FOR.

ISBN: 1-592-40081-7

Printed in the United States of America
Set in Adobe Garamond with Opti Archway Script and Flourish
Designed by Sabrina Bowers

To all the pregnant, soon-to-be pregnant, and recently pregnant women and couples who asked for this book. To all who so generously shared their experiences, you are the gold.

I especially dedicate this to the following moms and dads, who, with their soon-to-arrive babies, were with me literally step by step and month by month during the writing of Hot Mamas. *I wasn't kidding when I say everyone around me was pregnant.*

Billie & Dare, Debra & Emma, Mary Ann & Josephine, Michele & Sydney, Sandra & Maximillian, Maura & Cordell, Sophie & Dylan, Christian & Stella

Contents

Acknowledgments

There are many things about writing a book that are similar to being pregnant and having a baby. You are thrilled to first learn you will be creating one. You share your joy with your friends and then the impact of this event begins. You start a ten-month process that consumes your world. You don't remember when you weren't. And as you approach the delivery date, you wonder if you'll make the deadline and maybe, just maybe, you could extend it a bit, as there is more to do and prepare than you expected.

When I first shared with a novelist that I think of each book as a baby, his response was, "Lou, they are very much like having a child. You do as much as you can to prepare them for life, you protect them as best you can and, like children, you then send them out into the world, and only then do you see how they will touch other people's lives."

May the spirit of this child of mine bring you joy, make you laugh, and give you the gift of pleasure that others so generously shared with me.

This is where I get to thank all of the people who made this book possible. From my family and friends to peers and colleagues to those who had vision of its course when I didn't.

THE PERSONAL SUPPORT TEAM

Paul E. Nance . . . for all of the reasons you are in my life.

The fabulous women in my family, my sisters and nieces: Dede Paget-Dellio, Kathyrn Ireland, Sherry Paget, Michelle Paget, Lisa Paget,

Neilane Mayhew, and Tammy Kinghorn. I need another sisters' weekend soon.

My executive assistant Michele Thompson and her support team, Randy and Dustin Thompson.

Sherri Tenpenny, Sandra Beck, Maura McAniff, Jessica Kalkin, Frederick Goldencoat, Christian Thrasher, Sophie Biddle, Nicole Scheier, Nance Mitchell, Kendra King, Heather Shaw, Morley Winnick, Mike Friend and Randy Smith, Mark and Scott Charbonneau, Grace Evans, Eileen Michaels, Francisca Martinez, Priscilla Wallace, Jacqui Brandwynne, Jeff Harmon.

THE CREATIVE TEAM

Debra Goldstein, my fabulous agent. Dare I repeat it, you are an author's dream agent. Thank you again for your vision and support. And to your colleagues at The Creative Culture, Mary Ann Naples and Nicole Diamond Austin.

Billie Fitzpatrick, my writing collaborator—a woman who totally gets into her work. We delivered the final manuscript ten days before her daughter Dare arrived.

Lauren Marino, executive editor; Bill Shinker, publisher; Hilary Terrell, editorial assistant; and all at Gotham Books. Five times is the charm. It's so lovely to be working together again; you make this process easy.

Diego Felipe, illustrator; Donna Levine, copyeditor; Ray Lundgren, graphic artist for the cover.

Robin and Bob Park at Hollywood Webs for keeping me up and running.

THE RESEARCH AND DEVELOPMENT TEAM

Jules Black, M.D., Gil Mileikowsky, M.D., Karoline Bischof Guscetti, M.D., Ph.D., Sherri Tenpenny, D.O., Beverly Whipple, Ph.D., Patti Britton, Ph.D., Gary Richwald, M.D., Jacqui Snow, NP, MSC.

THE PRESENTATION TEAM

Lilianna and Ali Moradi, for their skill at keeping me presentable. Ron Derhacopian, again, for his stunning photography. Manuel Bonavides, an artist with a makeup brush.

Introduction

A GROUP OF WOMEN has gathered in the great room of a private residence for an evening—nothing new about that. There's also nothing new about the majority of these women being visibly pregnant. What is new is the subject they have gathered to discuss: sex during pregnancy.

Quite simply they are here to learn and share how being pregnant has changed and will likely change their sex lives. What can they expect? Will body parts, orgasms, and sexual relations ever be the same again? Unwilling to sit on the sidelines of life while they are pregnant, these women want to ensure that the intimate relationship that has created the babies they are now carrying doesn't vanish for the nine and a half months of gestation, or forever.

In the same way that I was asked to share the best information that women had shared with me in my internationally presented seminars and four bestselling books about all areas of sexuality (*How to Be a Great Lover, How to Give Her Absolute Pleasure, The Big O*, and *365 Days of Sensational Sex*), pregnant women have approached me, asking for the real goods on sexuality during pregnancy. They want honest, accurate, and candid information about what to expect in the beginning of the pregnancy, in the middle, at the end, and immediately after pregnancy because they have no intention of losing what has always been a crucially important part of their lives—their sexual selves. I call these women Hot Mamas.

Hot Mamas know only too well that pregnancy is now in its own social and cultural spotlight. Somewhere in the past decade, we woke up and realized that pregnancy can, in fact, be one of the most sensual, luscious times of a woman's life. After all, pregnant women are the ultimate earth mothers! We see them everywhere: beaming from the covers of magazines (sometimes in the nude), shopping at the chic boutiques that figured out that pregnancy and fashion are not mutually exclusive, and even accepting Academy Awards in zaftig style. The myth that pregnant women shouldn't or don't feel and look sexy has been blown out of the water thanks to countless Hot Mamas out there.

So why have these women approached me with their questions and desire to share? As a sex counselor with more than ten years' experience working in the field, a Certified Sex Educator, and a member of AASECT (American Association of Sex Educators, Counselors, and Therapists), I know how crucially important it is to provide information about sexuality that is accurate, age appropriate, and user-friendly. In the past ten years, as I have gathered more information and listened to thousands of women and men describe what works and doesn't work for them sexually, I began to notice that there has been a veritable baby boom going on. At one point every woman around me seemed to be pregnant—clients, friends, family . . . even my agent, writing partner, and executive assistant became pregnant at the same time. I was beginning to feel like an airborne pregnancy virus! (Not to suggest that pregnancy is a disease, of course.)

So, I created a new seminar especially for pregnant women and their partners. Most of the women who gather for these pregnancy seminars are already familiar with my attitude toward sexuality: that we are all born of sexuality, that there can't be anything more special than where we come from, and that we are all entitled to accurate, fun advice about sexuality that actually works. These women know they can rely on me to deliver information on all aspects of intimate relationships in an educated, safe, respectful, and nonjudgmental manner, enabling them to ask some of their most private questions.

They want to know more about what I have seen and heard in my seminars worldwide about how pregnancy and a new baby have affected many new parents' sex lives. What began as a few women and men asking such questions as "How do I keep things going sexually during pregnancy?"; "What do other couples do at seven months?"; "Will I feel the same for him?"; and "Do your parts change forever?" developed into a quest to gather information for these couples. These are the seeds from which this book grew.

Women who knew the joy and pleasure of their sexuality were not about to give it up just because they were pregnant. Yet they were frustrated because there was very little, if any, information out there that truly addressed sexuality during this most critically transformative time in a relationship. *Hot Mamas: The Ultimate Guide to Staying Sexy Throughout Your Pregnancy and the Months Beyond* is the result.

For me, Hot Mamas are the women who know intuitively that at no time in their lives is there likely to be a more pivotal point in their sexual relationship than during pregnancy. These women know "how to do it," "how to say it," and "how to keep it coming," so that despite the challenges of pregnancy (both physical and emotional), they stay sexually and/or sensually connected to themselves and their partners.

In no way does this book contain advice on what you should or should not do now that you are pregnant. Rather, *Hot Mamas* is about you and your partner finding a range of ideas and information so you can decide how you want to approach your sexuality during pregnancy. Unfortunately, the recent media coverage of celebrity moms has unwittingly created more pressure for women to do everything "right" during and after their pregnancies. And though most women want to do everything right, they want to do so within the context of what and how it is right *for them,* their baby, and their relationship. I know from experience that women know how to wade through the ocean of information out there, and, with shrewd female logic, they know that no one knows better about women's bodies than other women—especially when it comes to pregnancy. As a top ob-gyn told me, "Any woman who has been pregnant knows far more than a man could ever learn about pregnancy." By sharing the experiences of other pregnant couples, I am hoping that your own experiences will be informed, validated, and elucidated as you enter or re-enter this hugely complex and rewarding phase of life.

In addition to the expert advice of the many couples with whom I consulted, I have included *scientific explanations* to what so far have been only anecdotal reports of how women experience their sexuality during pregnancy. For example, why is it so many women are ripe and ready for more sex during pregnancy? Hormones. And the explanation is fairly straightforward. When not pregnant, many women can detect an increased sex drive during ovulation and during days 17–24. The reason behind these spikes in sexual appetite is directly related to the hormonal surges of estrogen and progesterone at these times in a woman's cycle. During pregnancy, women might jump to the conclusion that since they are not ovulating and not getting their menses, such spikes in libido would cease. However, pregnant women experience subtle yet real hormonal surges throughout their nine months of gestation that produce similar peaks in sexual desire.

Add to this sea of hormones a dramatic increase in blood volume. The result? Many pregnant women report experiencing an increase in the intensity of their orgasms. Since orgasms are naturally powered by blood, with each passing week and month of pregnancy, many women experience orgasms that are more and more intense as their blood volume increases by a total of 20 percent. Many times women have shared with me such remarks as "My pregnancy orgasms were the best of my life. They were vividly different from my nonpregnancy orgasms. I wish I could get to that place whenever I wanted!"

Some of my research is based on an online survey I conducted, which I sent to more than a hundred couples. In addition, and as I did in my previous books, I have garnered a *distinguished panel of medical experts* to provide the biological and scientific insight and support to further substantiate my own findings. Included among my panel of experts whose guidance and research I relied on are Jules Black, M.D.; Gil Mileikowsky, M.D.; Elizabeth Stewart, M.D.; Marc Ganem, M.D.; Kirsten von Sydow, Ph.D.; and Karoline Bischof, M.D., Ph.D. Both Dr. Black and Dr. Ganem are internationally renowned obstetrician gynecologists, as well as sexologists. Specifically, I've incorporated many of the findings from Dr. Ganem's invaluable book written in

French, *La Sexualité du couple pendant la grossesse* (*The Sexuality of Couples During Pregnancy*), which is based on his study of the sexuality of six hundred couples during pregnancy. In addition to numerous consultations, I've relied on thoughtful insight and provocative information gathered in Dr. Black's *Body Talk*, published in Australia and not available in the United States. Drs. von Sydow and Bischof have each written comprehensive research studies, from which I've pulled many interesting and valuable statistics and findings.

Hot Mamas is built around the four trimesters of pregnancy (the fourth trimester comprises the first six postpartum months). The book presents information about how pregnancy changes a woman emotionally, physically, and sexually. For each trimester, there is a chapter that addresses how to accept your body and adjust your attitude and your sex life so that you can experience the most pleasure—and peace of mind—possible.

Hot Mamas also reveals the stories, tips, and insights of the hundreds of women with whom I consulted, as well as those of many experts. For instance, you will:

- Find a whole new sexual dimension of yourself during pregnancy.
- Parlay your sexuality into sensuality in different ways during each trimester.
- Rediscover your anatomy. With the increased blood flow to your pelvis, your lower half will likely feel tighter and firmer, and you may never have felt so female or so erotic. You and your partner will learn new ways to tickle your fancy (and his, of course).
- Become a more sensual lover as you and your partner discover the ways you've changed: your sense of taste is different, your sense of smell is different, and how you experience touch is different. You will also learn some tricks for dealing with his natural male scent, which may now be off-putting to you.
- Learn how to redirect the very sensual and satisfying contact with your newborn into your sexual relationship with your partner. Once their new babies have arrived, many women realize that their interaction with their infants is very sensual and very

gratifying; sometimes, without being conscious of it, they sublimate *all* of their sensuality into caring for their babies, saving none of what could become the sensual and sexual desire with their partners. By becoming aware of this subtle but powerful shift in their attention, women can stay more sexually connected to their partners, as well as sensually connected with their infants.

▶ Be offered tips from women who never forgot the importance of having their partners know they remained a priority, despite pregnancy's maelstrom of physical and emotional changes. Such women always kept in mind that the whole reason they became mothers was because they were partners first.

▶ Choose your own timing for intimacy. As one client said to me, "It better happen before dinner or else I will have conked out. Now we've gotten really good at countertop sex."

▶ Be able to take advantage of your hormonal changes throughout your pregnancy. For example, the natural increase in oxytocin in your fourth trimester will increase your snuggle factor but may inhibit your libido.

It is my hope that once you read about the hundreds of women with whom I've spoken, you will feel more free to explore your own sexuality during and after pregnancy. I feel any pregnant woman should give herself permission to feel sexy, be sexy, ask questions, and learn techniques, and also the freedom to decide how she wants to experience her own pregnancy. The women who wear the Hot Mama banner think of themselves as future mothers and as sexual beings. They do not separate these important roles, although culturally the two so often become separated in our minds, which is ironic, since sex is what led to pregnancy in the first place! As you explore your changing body, you may find that, in spite of intense fatigue and growing ungainliness, you are a remarkably versatile sexual being. I have also included the male view of pregnancy. It is clear that men, too, want to have more permission to be involved in every aspect of a woman's pregnancy. Men today are challenging the dyad of mother and child and want to be included, which is not only more fun for all involved, it's also more healthy for the entire family. But men also remain stymied by unnecessary doubts, myths, and often a stubborn feeling or fear of being excluded from the pregnancy.

Here's the bottom line: pregnancy can be one of the sauciest, sexiest times of a woman's life, and it is time that women everywhere be given the validation, the information, and the awareness to make this happen should they decide they want the rewards of a sexually vital pregnancy.

Hot Mamas

The First Trimester

Sex During Pregnancy:
The Challenges and the Payoffs

LADIES, I AM HERE TO SHARE with you how other couples have benefited physically, emotionally, and spiritually by keeping their sexual pilot lights on during pregnancy. It's entirely up to you to choose when and how to turn on the heat, but by listening and staying open to the experience of others, you may feel more informed and therefore more motivated to remain sexual throughout your pregnancy. Consider what Colleen, a forty-year-old mother, shared with me: "This is my second pregnancy, and I seem to have no recollection of ever feeling this tired with my first child. But this one has really taken the wind out of my sails. Usually my partner and I have sex once or twice a week—sometimes even three times. But once I started getting so tired, I just didn't feel like sex. Then we tried it—what can I say? It's like a magic elixir—the sex makes me feel more energetic and less tired!"

Now, before you begin to mentally fling items at Colleen, let me assure you that Colleen is not alone. Nicole, a university law professor, shared, "I developed an entirely different relationship with exhaustion. I now know the meaning of bone weary. Yet exhausted as I was, I still found my husband hot. When I got home from work, all I wanted was to be held by him. Call me crazy, but staying sexual with him was what took care of me." It's true: sex during pregnancy not only happens but it can also deliver enormous pleasure, gratification, and sometimes welcome relief.

However, lest you think I have heard only one perspective—not so. I spoke with plenty of women who said they were not at all interested in sex during pregnancy. "You've got to be kidding," said Mariellen when I asked her if she experienced an increase in her libido during pregnancy. "I wouldn't let my husband near me! I was so exhausted and so sick during my first three months, sex was the furthest thing from my mind." But after a thoughtful pause, she added, "It's been almost two years, and I wish I had stayed sexual with my husband. But it was like society gave me an excuse—you don't hear a lot about pregnant women wanting or needing sex. I just thought it was natural to stop, so I didn't even try."

Other women also expressed their regret about not having stayed sexually connected to their partners during pregnancy. Dana said, "Sex was the last thing I wanted. I felt so weighed down physically and emotionally, I just wanted to be left alone. But now I see how long it has taken to get our relationship back on the sexual track."

The deep frustration of these women came through loud and clear. At the time, they didn't feel the motivation to be sexual, but they also never considered choosing to be sexual. As a result, they often felt alone and overwhelmed by their lack of connection to their partners— not exactly an inspired mood for sex. So how can women respond differently to this situation? Is there a way to get in the mood when the challenges of pregnancy seem stacked against you?

From listening to hundreds of women who did stay sexually connected—to themselves and their partners—during their first trimesters and throughout their pregnancies, I found that the consistent underlying factor was their having made a conscious decision to be and stay sexual. The women who enjoyed sexual and sensual pleasure throughout the tumultuous nine and a half months also held fast to a common belief: that the best thing they could do for themselves, their relationship, and the future well-being of their soon-to-be-born child was to stay in touch with that part of themselves that allowed sexual pleasure and sought out fulfillment of that desire.

This chapter is devoted to looking at what's going on with you emotionally and psychologically during your first trimester so that you can consider making the choice to stay sexually and sensually alive during your first trimester and throughout your pregnancy. How you approach and handle your sexuality is up to you. It's a private, personal decision that requires thought and care. And while I respect any choice or decision made, I do want to add one insight I've learned from working with thousands of women, men, and couples over my twelve-year career in sexuality: the more women stay open to their sexuality—in its many guises—the stronger and more self-assured they feel in every aspect of their lives, pregnant or not.

The Reality of Staying Sexually Connected During Pregnancy

There is no doubt that pregnancy is one of the most challenging times of a woman's life. The mental and emotional shift that is taking place can be quite dramatic. Along with your expanding waistline and the hundreds of other biological changes that are going on, you are probably mentally grappling with the whole idea of changing your life forever by becoming a mother. Indeed, there can be many things rather frightening about moving into motherhood. In a 1999 study presented to the annual clinical meeting of the Society of Obstetricians and Gynecologists, Dr. Elias Bartellas, professor at the Memorial University of Newfoundland, reported that more than 42 percent of 142 pregnant women surveyed revealed that their sexual desire was either the same or increased during pregnancy. This finding was reinforced by my own survey of 30 couples in which 41.6 percent (12) of the women who responded said they experienced an increase in their libido and sex drive.

What do these numbers mean?

Quite simply, they show that about 58 percent of women feel sexually encumbered by the challenges of pregnancy. They are either so uncomfortable with the physical and emotional changes brought on by pregnancy that they lose touch with their libido, or they are reluctant and afraid to see themselves as sexual beings while preparing for motherhood. But before you feel too demoralized to read further or too disconnected from such experiences, let me present another interesting finding. In an even more recent metacontent analysis study, in which Dr. Kirsten von Sydow analyzed the findings of fifty-nine studies conducted between 1950 and 1996 of sexuality during pregnancy and after childbirth, it was found that though "on average, female sexual interest and coital activity declines slightly in the first trimester . . . 82 percent of a female sample think that intercourse should be practiced during the whole pregnancy. When intercourse must be avoided for medical reasons, 82 percent prefer mutual petting."

These numbers don't contradict the study mentioned above, but instead point to how complicated pregnancy and sex is for many women. If only 42 percent of women reported feeling in touch with their libido but 82 percent know it's best to stay sexually connected to themselves and their partners during pregnancy, then there is a discrepancy between what women want and what women experience. I'd like to focus on making all 82 percent not only desirous of being sexual but capable and fulfilled by doing so. The slightly smaller group of women (the 42 percent) show that it is possible to feel not only sexually turned on during this time but motivated to stay sexually aware and connected to oneself and one's partner—despite the challenges presented by pregnancy.

This premise is further supported by Dr. von Sydow's findings that "if both partners are sexually active during pregnancy and enjoy it, the relationship is evaluated as better with regard to tenderness and communication at four months postpartum, and three years later, the relationship is more stable and less affected in the view of both partners." That is the ultimate promise of staying sexual throughout one's pregnancy: by staying sexually connected during this time, you make sure that you can take care of your child, yourself, and your relationship.

So how do you make the choice to stay sexually connected during your first trimester and throughout your pregnancy?

The Hot Mama Attitude
(or Making the Choice to Be a Hot Mama)

In talking with hundreds of people, I found that one of the biggest challenges for most pregnant women and couples is experienced in the area of attitude. How does a pregnant woman get in touch with the deep roots of her sexual desire if she is feeling overwhelmed and vulnerable? How does she stay in touch with her sensuality when she feels physically tired and moody? In many ways, the first trimester is the most challenging of all four trimesters of pregnancy. Even though you are barely showing, your body and mind are going through their most intense changes during the first twelve weeks of pregnancy. (I will go into the physical nature of these first-trimester changes in the next chapter.) And yet, despite these very real challenges, some women found that the earlier they adopted a Hot Mama attitude, the more they benefited over the subsequent six and a half months of pregnancy.

So what is a Hot Mama? First let me describe her. She walks with confidence, knowing that she is in possession of the ultimate power: the ability to create life. She happily accepts the warm smiles sent her way from strangers as she makes her way through her day, absorbing the accolades and happy sentiments from the world into the core of her being. She eats nourishing food that makes her skin glow. She exercises to whatever degree she can to keep her energy up and her body in shape. And most of all, she stays deeply connected to her innate sensual and sexual nature. In essence, a Hot Mama is a woman who takes care of herself.

This commitment to herself is just as much an attitude as it is a set of behaviors. For as much as Hot Mamas try to eat the right things, get exercise, pay attention to their men and their relationships, they also give themselves breaks—whenever they need them. As Mary Kate so aptly put it, "I gave myself plenty of room to grow—and by grow I don't mean physically, I mean emotionally. I just stayed open to how my body was changing and didn't fight it. I wanted to enjoy the experience as much as possible. I mean, I had a baby growing inside of me!"

Hot Mamas know intuitively that sexuality and pregnancy are two of the most highly charged experiences of their lives and as such can give women access to a deep strength within themselves. This strength is not a static, cold, or bracing power, but rather a pliable resilience and the ability to adapt to their present reality—in this case, pregnancy. When women stay open, soft, and receptive to their transforming bodies, hearts, and minds—all of which change because of pregnancy—they are then able to stay connected to all parts of themselves, including their sexuality. This connection is vital to a woman's continued ability and motivation to take care of herself. When pregnant women tap into this lush source of strength, they tap into the deepest level of self-care. For I believe that no woman can be truly happy, or be a good lover, partner, or mother, if she does not first learn how to take care of herself—body and soul. This is the essence of being a Hot Mama.

By taking care of herself, a Hot Mama builds confidence in all areas of her life, including managing the highs and lows of pregnancy, staying involved in her relationship, and preparing for the arrival of her baby. Further, many women I spoke with declared that on the way to motherhood, they actually felt more sexually confident. Why? Their reasons varied, but here is a sampling:

- They felt more empowered physically. Witnessing their bodies go through pregnancy put them more in touch with their bodies' strength and abilities, which in turn helped them feel more in touch with their sexual power.
- They discovered an entirely new and different way to feel and be sexy. No longer in competition with the glossy magazine shots of Jessica Simpson and Angelina Jolie, some of the pregnant women with whom I spoke said they felt sexier than ever because they felt less encumbered by how others define "sexy." As one woman captured it, "I became the original earth woman—come to me, baby, let me show you how it's done!"
- They became more forgiving of their bodies' imperfections and more focused on how much pleasure their bodies actually gave them during pregnancy!

As Carly said, "My big breasts made me feel sexy, and I found my big belly to be very erotic—an opinion my husband shared." Susan said, "I was surprised that I felt so sexy and that I still wanted to make love. It also helped that my partner was very turned on by my body's changes." The underlying premise of being a Hot Mama in both attitude and behavior is sexual confidence—the confidence to accept your body and its limitations, explore new sexual territory with your partner, and embrace your pregnant self.

The bottom line here, ladies, is that you too can be a Hot Mama. You can rise to the occasion and its challenges, embracing your curves and the burgeoning sexuality that can grow right along with your belly. All it takes is that you choose to adopt an attitude of

- ➤ openness and willingness
- ➤ adaptability and resilience
- ➤ acceptance and flexibility

With this frame of mind in place, your strength and confidence will grow, supporting you through the long haul and motivating you to seek out pleasure and enjoyment when you want to. It's all up to you.

Hot Mama vs. Fat-n-Frumpy

At the very moment you know you're pregnant, you have a choice: you can put in the time and effort to remain a Hot Mama, or you can slide down the slippery slope of self-neglect and become what some women affectionately call a Fat-n-Frumpy.

You know the Fat-n-Frumpies. They are the women who constantly look miserable, swathed in unflattering layers of oversized clothes. They not only look nauseated all the time, but make sure to tell anyone within earshot how many times they threw up that day. Cut off from the neck down, they balloon to sometimes dangerous weights almost immediately, believing they have license to let themselves go completely. More often than not, these are the women whose relationships come to a stalemate. Ask them if they feel sexy while pregnant, and they are likely to glare at you as though you were nuts. But what makes a pregnant woman a Fat-n-Frumpy rather than a Hot Mama comes down to attitude. The attitude of a Fat-n-Frumpy is what makes these women feel unattractive. Let's be serious, I have seen very large, two hundred pounds+ size women who look awesome, and women who have gained a mere twenty-two pounds who look and feel miserable. It's all a matter of outlook and choice.

Stay In Touch with Who You Are

Just because you're pregnant does not mean that you have to shed your personality as if you were awaiting a virgin birth. Indeed, from what I have gathered from the hundreds of women with whom I consulted for this book, those who enjoyed their pregnancy the most, including an enjoyment of their carnal nature, were those women who continued doing what they liked to do—whether taking a Pilates class, lunching with friends, shopping, or holing up and reading a book—for as long as they could. They made themselves feel as normal and grounded as possible as they entered this dramatic nine-and-a-half-month period of change.

A lot of women told me that one of the best ways to stay connected to oneself during pregnancy is to keep working, assuming you did so before you got pregnant. Robyn, a financial planner who became pregnant for the first time at thirty-four, found that her job was the one thing she knew she could count on to make her feel like herself during those nine months. "Almost as soon as I found out I was pregnant, my whole world felt like it got turned upside down," she said. "My body was going through all these bizarre and unsettling changes—even coffee tasted weird!—but the one thing that really kept me feeling grounded was going to work. I love my job, and something about continuing to be effective in the world was very steadying. In the middle of all the chaos going on in my body, at least I knew my business sense was still going strong!"

Keying in to your sensuality at this early stage is another way to stay connected to yourself as you slowly but surely integrate the knowledge of your impending motherhood. By staying sensually alert, these pregnant women kept themselves more open to experiencing their sexual feelings. As Petra said, "I can't say I felt particularly sexual—especially during my first trimester—but I did take care of my body. I wanted to look good and feel good. That was so important to me."

There are so many small choices you can make every single day that can keep you feeling good, fresh, and attractive. Here are some suggestions other pregnant women have used to keep themselves feeling good during pregnancy:

- Shave your legs (for as long as you can still see them).
- Get a really good haircut to accentuate your fabulous, glossy new tresses.
- Fight the urge to eat everything in your path, remembering that no one feels good seventy pounds over their normal weight and that what you eat affects how you feel.
- Trim those Teflon-strong new nails with regular manicures and pedicures.
- Gloss those big, luscious lips. Even when—no, *especially* when—you feel too tired to do so.
- Have lunch with your girlfriends, even if it's just a take-out salad.
- Don't miss your yoga class or other regular exercise.

The take-home message here is: do whatever it takes to feel normal, invigorated, and good about yourself.

And if this is not your first pregnancy, then review what you liked and didn't like about previous pregnancies—now is the time to make a change, especially one in attitude. As one woman said of her second pregnancy, "During my first pregnancy I was nervous—I stopped exercising, withdrew sensually and sexually from my partner. But this time I simply refused to deny myself all that pleasure, and I knew that it would actually be better for the baby. So I remained as active as I could and barely strayed from my normal routine until the third trimester. That made a big difference in how I felt!"

Stay Connected to Him

Many women experience an emotional shutdown in their first trimester because so much is happening inside their bodies. Anxious and nervous about this waiting period, distracted by the possibility of a miscarriage (85 percent of all miscarriages happen in the first trimester and are unrelated to any actions of the mother—see pages 32–33 for further information), many women clam up—verbally and sexually—especially with the ones who matter the most, their partners. Women have said again and again that what they found most important during these early months of pregnancy was knowing their men were available and attentive. Indeed, Dr. Marc Ganem said that to enjoy their pregnancies, women need three things:

- ➤ affection
- ➤ protection
- ➤ love

Yet women cannot assume their partners know of these three needs. Instead, they need to articulate what they need and want from their partners so their partners can then have a chance to quell their fears. One of the best things you can do is keep talking. Though you want to control your feelings by bottling them up inside, let them out and share them with your partner. The more he knows about your feelings, the more likely it is that he will be there for you. This comfort will feel reassuring.

Some of the women I spoke with shared that one of their first worries when they learned they were pregnant was that their husbands or partners would suddenly disappear. And although these women admitted that that was unlikely, the fear remained. The antidote? Loving partners who were physically present—be it caressing, comforting, or making love to them. From my research I learned that staying connected to your partner—either sensually or sexually—will lessen the likelihood that you will feel isolated, vulnerable, and alone. Indeed, the more you stay connected to your man, the more support and comfort you will feel and the more inspired your attitude will be.

Staying emotionally connected to your partner during pregnancy benefits not only your well-being but also your relationship. As Kerry, age thirty-nine, said, "My relationship with Michael was my lifeline. Everything was changing—my body, my future, how I lived my day-to-day life. I needed him more than ever. But the most amazing thing I discovered was that he needed me, too."

And remember, as all-encompassing as pregnancy is for you, men have their own intense experience of it as well. When I asked Michael (Kerry's husband) how he felt during Kerry's pregnancy, he said, "I wanted desperately to be a part of the process. I was so afraid of her shutting me out—not just from sex but from all of her. So even when she was exhausted, I would just try to comfort her. I would bring her hot tea, rub her feet, do errands for her—anything to show her how much I cared."

Your man needs to know (and therefore be told) that the most important thing he can do for you is to be there for you, reassuring you during your first trimester. With so many things changing and seeming out of your control, you want him to let you know that he is more than interested in sticking around. While this fear may seem irrational, it can be very real for some women—but you cannot assume men get this automatically or psychically.

But keep in mind that communicating is not complaining. Another fear many men experience when their partners become pregnant is that the women will become large complainers. As one gentleman in his late thirties admitted, "When my wife got pregnant with our second child, all I could think about was how she was going to whine for the next nine months." When I asked him if his wife had complained a lot during her first pregnancy, he said, "Well, no. Not at all. But—" And when I queried, "But what?" he said, "But I was afraid she would."

My point, ladies? Sharing your state of mind, your state of body, and your state of spirit with your man does not require a whiny, complaining voice. Indeed, he will become an even better listener if he hears you directly. Here are a few small tips from someone who speaks with and listens to men worldwide:

- Always be as clear as you can; try to say it in one sentence.
- Deliver one subject at a time.
- Be as nonjudgmental as you can, as he can't know what you are going through.

So keep talking to each other. Share the information you are learning about your pregnancy, tell him you need and want him, and respect his needs and experience, too. It always takes two to tango.

What Men Have Said About Their Women During Pregnancy

The results from my online survey were very clear: one of the most important factors for women staying sexual during their pregnancy was knowing that their partners still found them attractive. Here are a few lines that should make you purr inside:

- "I was in awe of how her body kept changing; I couldn't get enough of her."

- "The way her hips spread gave her ass an exaggerated heart shape, which drove me nuts."
- "I had moments when I wished I were a woman—just a moment, of course. And then I would just attach myself to my wife and try to become part of her—it was all very intense."
- "She was so sick and I just wanted to help her feel better, and one thing I did do was I held her hair while she threw up."
- "I thought maybe watching her give birth would somehow affect how I looked at her sexually, but it wasn't like that at all. I just looked at her in wonder."
- "I'm a real wuss when it comes to body stuff so we knew from the start I would stay close to her head and comfort her that way."

Plan Sex

How do you make your mind transcend matter? How do you find the time and energy to have sex with your man when you are busy—with work, kids, or work and kids—and can't seem to fit even a twenty-minute break into your schedule? You plan it. You're worth it.

Planning sex is no less important than planning all the other events in your life—work meetings, doctor appointments, birthday parties for children, and family get-togethers. For such events to take place, you need to make time and plan them. It's that simple, and the same applies to sex.

I've written several other books that mention the importance of organizing and planning for sex, but the circumstances of pregnancy make this step even more imperative. Planning sex doesn't have to be elaborate. Connecting sexually can mean snuggling for two hours or an uninterrupted meal during which you don't talk about children but instead talk about you and your future together.

Here are some suggestions:

- If you have children, hire a baby-sitter and send them to the zoo or on some sort of outing. In other words, figure out a way for you and your husband to have the entire house to yourselves for at least two hours, even if it's just for sleeping.
- If you don't have children but are otherwise too tired and busy to set aside time for passion, then you need to put it on your calendar or in your PDA or cell phone—just like all the other activities to which you commit. Take a tip from my friend Kendra: avoid planning sex on Friday nights, because by then you might be too tired. Instead, try for a midweek break, such as a Tuesday or a Wednesday evening.
- If your primary impediment seems to be morning sickness or nausea, consider a couple of the remedies other women have used (see page 43), and then schedule a calm, erotic interlude with your partner afterward.
- The bottom line: try to connect—either sexually or sensually— at least once a week with your husband or partner.

The point here is about your intention to stay intimate with your partner. There may well be times when you are just not in the mood, even though you have planned a sexual encounter. But rather than turn away from each other when plans go awry—for whatever reason— continue to remind yourself of your intention to stay close. As Lotita said, "We cuddled more and in some ways felt even closer than before I got pregnant. It was nice not to always assume sex meant intercourse." At times like this, the definition of great sex is between you and your partner, and that means giving yourselves the permission to explore and accept wherever your sexual road may lead at that time.

Making Sex Fun Again

In this age of fertility treatments and many women waiting longer to have children, some women have told me that it was difficult to think about sex as being fun once they were pregnant. "Because it took us so long to get pregnant—almost four years of trying, with the injections and the seemingly endless waiting periods between attempts—sex had become so mechanical. Once we were pregnant, all we felt was relieved that we didn't have to have sex again." Why wouldn't you and your partner feel relief if sex had become such a chore, separated from fun and passion? It only makes sense. Now it's time to find that fun factor again.

First, you need to refresh your attitude: your mission has been accomplished (you're pregnant), and sex is no longer work. It's meant to be fun, pleasurable, and passionate, and it can be—even when you're pregnant. When you and your partner focus on this changed perspective, your sex life will lose the work flavor and feel much more like those heady days of passion you shared when you were first together.

Next, you need to review your sexual history with your partner and remind yourselves of what you enjoyed sexually before sex began to feel like work. Now is the time to mine those memory banks for tried-and-true techniques to get you both in the mood. (You may also want to skip ahead two chapters and find some ideas to wet your whistle, and his.)

Here are a few tips to help you delve into your reservoirs of fun and passion:

- Cultivate the deliciousness of having a secret. For those of you who have elected not to share your news with anyone until you are in your second trimester, relishing your privacy can be a rich way of brewing passion between the two of you. The intimacy of this special secret will bring you closer—in mind, body, and spirit.
- Plan fun encounters. Don't wait for the mood to strike you: plan a seduction or some other sexual encounter that you know will excite both of you.
- Plan two or three pre-baby escape "babymoons" where you can concentrate on all parts of you and your relationship—away from the buzz of day-to-day responsibilities and obligations.

Exercise:
A Key to Taking Care of Yourself

Exercise not only helps you stay physically fit; it helps you stay emotionally fit. This may sound like a giant cliché, but it's absolutely true and more important than ever now that you are pregnant. Staying physically fit and strong increases your ability to experience sexual and sensual pleasure throughout your pregnancy. But even more important is how exercise keeps you feeling good about yourself, which is key to feeling like a Hot Mama. As Grace said, "I didn't have to do much— maybe take a walk with a friend or do twenty minutes on my husband's stationary bike. But I felt so much better—the least amount of exercise made me feel pumped up and happy." Other clients said that exercise not only quelled any morning sickness but also made them feel better—less tired and more energetic. Barbara remembered that "the more I ran, the better I felt. It was like the blood ran faster through my veins—and that feeling definitely made me feel more like myself, and I wanted to have sex!"

Beyond the lift exercise can give your spirits, there are many other benefits of continuing to stay active throughout your pregnancy. As Peter Nathanielsz, M.D., Ph.D., points out in his book *The Prenatal Prescription,* the benefits are manifold:

- Women have more energy during pregnancy.
- Women gain less weight during pregnancy and stay within the limits for a healthy weight gain.
- Women report fewer instances of discomfort due to pregnancy and during labor.
- Labor tends to be shorter for women who have continued exercising.
- Women feel better, have more energy, and feel more optimistic.

Exercise also benefits the baby:

- There are fewer incidents of meconium in the amniotic fluid, a sign of fetal stress.
- Babies of mothers who exercise tend to quiet themselves more easily, which is related to a "toned-down stress response system."

But the best advice during your pregnancy is to keep in mind the benefits of continuing exercise for the sake of your sexual pleasure quotient. My expert sources as well as my many clients say that staying as active as possible during pregnancy helps offset all the negative physical symptoms and makes them feel more open to being sexual. Also, the more fit you are, the more relaxed you will feel, which will increase your chances of being in the mood for sex. After exercise your body may feel tired, but you have pumped up your body with a neurohormone called beta-endorphin that will help improve your mood. We've all heard of the "runner's high," and what is sex but one of Mother Nature's most natural forms of exercise!

KEGELS

There is one particular exercise that gets right to the heart of sexual pleasure: Kegels. Kegels strengthen and tone the pubococcygeus muscle (PC muscle), which runs from the front to the back of the pelvic girdle like a hammock. For women during pregnancy, the weight of the baby stretches these bands of muscle, making them less effective in their function for bladder control. Another PC muscle function is to contract rhythmically during orgasm. This little muscle gives the telltale quivers and contractions of orgasm that occur at 0.8 per second. Gentlemen also have a PC muscle, which is responsible for the "jumps" an erect penis makes.

Kegels and the Pelvic Floor

The more you strengthen and tone your PC muscle, the more likely you will orgasm, and the greater the intensity. And the more you engage your pelvic floor muscles, in general, the more sexual enjoyment you will be able to experience.

DETERMINE THE STRENGTH OF YOUR PC MUSCLE

Before beginning your Kegels, determine the strength of your PC muscle by inserting your index and middle fingers into your vagina and squeezing around them as if you were trying to stop the flow of urine. Most women need to use two fingers, as one isn't thick enough. The exercising motion for the PC is identical to that of stopping the flow of urine. Contract firmly around your fingers. If the band of pressure feels like a thin line, you need to do some work. If it feels broad, then your PC is in decent shape—but like all our muscles, it can probably benefit from some toning.

HOW TO DO KEGELS

This is a small muscle group, so you can fatigue them easily. Here's how to get started:

1. Contract your PC muscle from the entry of your vagina back toward your anus. You can think of this in two ways: imagine you are squeezing your partner's penis, or imagine that you are trying to stop the flow of urine.

2. Start by holding the contraction tightly for five seconds, and then release for five seconds. Repeat this sequence for a few

minutes up to five times daily, gradually increasing the time for each set five minutes. Another variation recommended by Dr. Black, one of my expert consultants, is to try to build up to doing roughly two hundred Kegels per day, doing ten sets of twenty.

3. For best results, pull in your PC muscle all the way for five to ten seconds and then release. Don't make the mistake of caving your stomach in and contracting at the belly button level. Those are abdominal contractions, not PC contractions.

4. Some women practice their Kegels by clenching a tampon as they remove it.

5. For more variety, practice flutters (quick contractions of one to two seconds).

Women have become very creative at fitting Kegels into their daily routine. One woman used to practice her Kegels while urinating. "As soon as I started the flow, I'd hold until it stopped. Sometimes it took me five minutes to go to the bathroom, but the result was worth it." Another woman, a mother of four, said she does her Kegels in the car. "I spend more than half my day schlepping my kids around town, so now I do my Kegels at every stop sign." And yet another woman does her Kegels while brushing her teeth.

There are also a few devices that help create more resistance and awareness of your PC muscle as you do your Kegels, including the Vaginal Weight-Lifting Eggs, the Kegelcisor, and the more ergonomically designed Energie™. The Kegelcisor is a silver-plated metal device used to exercise a woman's PC muscle. It looks like a barbell and is approximately six inches long and three-quarters of an inch in diameter. There are two enlarged, rounded ends and a smooth, centrally raised "donut" in the middle. It works very simply: with both the Kegelcisor and the Energie™, the woman assumes a reclining position, gently inserts one end of the Kegelcisor into her well-lubricated vagina and squeezes as she would during a Kegel. Because of the solidness and weight (14 oz; 400g) of the object, a woman can contract her PC muscle with more resistance and awareness. Some women find they prefer to support the external portion of these exercisers, as it helps them focus on the contractions.

For those women who prefer a vertical exercising position, Vaginal Weight-Lifting Eggs are an ideal way to tone and firm your PC muscle while standing or walking. Gravity's natural tendency to have the egg slip out helps to sensitize the PC muscle that it has something to hold in place. Made of polished onyx the size of a large egg, it works by having a solid item the PC muscle can be aware of and contract around. Weighing approximately three to five ounces, the egg is inserted by a woman fully into her vagina. Some women use a lubricant while others do not, and some warm the egg with warm water while others prefer the cool sensation of the onyx as it is inserted. A woman can walk around with the egg in place while flexing her PC muscles, or she can stand in place and do repeated, focused PC muscle contractions while letting the egg drop and then contracting firmly to move it back up the vaginal vault. The egg is removed like a tampon by a gently pulling on an attached nylon string.

The *fria*™ is a device that contains a computerized chip program, a monitor, and an insertable vaginal wand that measures the intensity of your contractions. You contract around a small ballooned wand with sensors inside that allow you to easily follow the guided PC exercise program on the monitor's screen while getting immediate feedback on the intensity of your contractions.

MORE EXERCISE TIPS

You may be one of those pregnant women to whom no exercise seems to appeal. As Carla said, "I couldn't even bend my head forward—I would feel dizzy or nauseous with any movement." Obviously, if something doesn't feel good, then don't do it.

Aside from Kegels, here are some more tips for staying active during your pregnancy:

➤ Walk, walk, walk.
➤ Practice yoga, Pilates, or other exercises that combine stretching, resistance training, and your mind-body connection.

➤ Do light weight training, especially for your arms.

➤ Perform deep squats: keeping your legs parallel and as wide as a yoga mat, begin with ten squats and work toward twenty-five.

➤ Do pelvic tilts: lying on your back with your knees bent, raise your fanny off the floor. Keep as much of your back on the floor as possible, focusing on lifting your fanny.

In the chapters ahead, I will be offering more specific tips on exercises that strengthen your body while increasing your potential for experiencing sexual pleasure. Keep these general suggestions in mind for now and continue doing what you've been doing. And remember, pay attention to your body and honor where it is right now. If you need to relax and rest, then do that. If you wake up and feel energetic, then get some exercise—take advantage of this surge. If you wake up feeling tired and worn out, then rest. Give yourself the day off or the week off. Know that the more you give your body what it needs, the more it will give back to you.

Exercise Common Sense

Now is not the time to start something new. The general rule of thumb for exercise during pregnancy is to continue what you're used to doing. As Dr. Black recommends, "If you can still talk while exercising, you're fine. But if you get breathless, then you need to slow down."

Making Your Intention Real

Being sexual at any time during our lives is a conscious decision. Being sexual throughout your pregnancy is a bigger conscious decision, as there are many things that can and will interrupt your intimacy. I repeat the following not as a judgment but so you are aware: if you don't clearly and consciously intend to have sex, then you will probably end up falling into the chasm of a chaste pregnancy. Not only is this chasm like quicksand—hard to get out of—it also precludes the emotional and spiritual connection your sex life has the promise to deliver.

Indeed, if you are open to the possibility and willing to try, then you just may surprise your very tired self. You may find that with a little self-induced push and some encouragement from your no doubt able and willing partner, you can overcome your fatigue and find sexual pleasure. It's not only possible, it's entirely probable—but you have to do three things:

1. Have the intention.

2. Try it.

3. Push the envelope.

This is the essence of being a Hot Mama.

And as soon as you decide to be a Hot Mama, you have to be ready to act. As you try to make the conscious decision to stay sexually active and connected to yourself and your partner throughout your pregnancy, you must be willing to experiment. Try a new position. Introduce some manual play you otherwise relegate to the foreplay of yesteryear. Continue to connect with your partner in all ways—physical, emotional, spiritual, and sexual. And finally, harness the wonderful, energized confidence of a Hot Mama and push the sexual envelope by moving beyond your own boundaries and expectations of pleasure. When you become an explorer instead of a passive observer of your pregnancy, you open yourself (and your lucky partner!) to marvels of intimacy only imagined.

In the pages ahead, you will find many ways to get in the mood (and stay) and be sexual and sensual throughout your pregnancy. Let these ideas entice you, encourage you, and perhaps at times challenge you to remain sexual and/or sensual. Do what feels good for you and your partner. And while I don't often resort to scare tactics, I do want to pass on this tidbit of information: the mutual happiness of couples can decrease markedly after the birth of their first child. As Kirsten von Sydow states, "The sexual relationship seems to be the most vulnerable area in the relationship of expectant and young parents."

So, ladies, the challenge and benefits are yours. You have the information, and you know what attitude works. Now you need to push that sexual envelope, trusting that the other side will deliver not only great sexual pleasure but also a passion and a connection with your partner you heretofore could only fantasize about.

In the next chapter, you will be able to gather more information about the inner and outer changes your body is undergoing in the first trimester of pregnancy. While some of these changes may be all too familiar to you, you will see them in the light of their impact on your sexuality.

2

Internal Shifts, External Vibrations
Stage One of Your Changing Body

REMEMBER THAT EMOTIONAL ROLLER COASTER I spoke of? The reasons behind it are largely physiological in nature. Are you one of the hundreds of women who go through "hormone hell" during their first trimester, subject to bends, dips, and peaks of mood and energy? Are your breasts too tender to even wear a bra comfortably? Is nausea a 24/7 thing for you? (Take heart: it should abate at about sixteen weeks.) Do you feel so chilled you cannot seem to ever get warm? Are you so tired you want to go to bed at six P.M.? Many women feel their most fatigued during the first trimester: Sharon told me it was a good thing she worked from home because she would literally fall asleep over her computer. And before they even know that they're pregnant, some women may wonder about the hypersensitivity in their breasts and vagina, or that extra juiciness between their legs. Others feel so nauseated they wish they could wake up in nine months. So how can you and your partner not only get in the mood but stay in the mood for sex?

These are very real challenges to having sex at all during your initial three months of pregnancy, let alone good sex. As Patricia shared with me, the motto for this trimester should be "This too shall pass." And while there is no doubt that your nausea, breast tenderness, and fatigue make getting in the mood rather daunting, there is nothing physical that should impede sex during this trimester if your medical professional has told you that you are having a normal pregnancy. Indeed, you may feel more comfortable making the choice to stay sensually and/or sexually active if you have a better sense of what is going on inside that growing body of yours. Let's take a closer look at how you are changing, so that you are better able and prepared to deal with the effects of those changes outside of your body.

Hormonal Shifts and Increases

Although externally it may seem like little has changed with your body in these first twelve weeks of pregnancy, internally, your body is moving into high gear. These internal changes are fueled by a release of a number of hormones, each having its own function for ensuring the proper implantation of your fetus; the growth of the placenta, which will sustain the fetus; the preparation of your body for the nine months ahead; and the protection and safe arrival of both you and your baby on the other end of this nine-month journey. Aside from their important role in organogenesis (the growth of the organs of your fetus), these hormones also play a role in your sexuality. Indeed, as I stated in the Introduction, pregnancy can increase your libido, and this is largely due to increased hormonal activity. Here is a breakdown of how these powerful hormones affect your body and your sexuality in the first trimester:

➤ The increase in **estrogen** circulating in the body is swift and dramatic. The amount of estrogen produced in a single day is equivalent to that generated by a nonpregnant woman's ovaries in three years. During the course of a single pregnancy, a woman produces as much estrogen as a nonpregnant woman could over 150 years. Many women respond to this increase in estrogen with a heightened libido.

➤ **Estrogen** also fosters a sense of well-being, as well as shining hair, supple and glowing skin, and an aura of tranquility and contentment—all of which contribute to a woman's ability to be relaxed for and receptive to sex.

- The placenta produces **testosterone,** which enters the mother's bloodstream, increasing her libido. Researchers are finding that pregnant women experience subtle yet very real hormonal surges throughout their nine months of gestation that produce similar peaks of sexual desire.

- To grow the placenta, the level of **progesterone** rises to ten times what it was before conception. Progesterone's main role is to protect against the mother's body's rejecting the fetus as a foreign body. It is also linked to the slowing down of your digestive system, as it works on the smooth muscle tissue of the organs involved. Sexually, this means that some women may take longer to orgasm.

- As soon as your placenta starts to grow, the body releases an increased amount of **relaxin**. Like it sounds, relaxin literally relaxes the ligaments of the body as a way to prepare it for labor and delivery. Since one of the roles of this hormone is to soften the pelvic girdle, many women find themselves physically more soft and open during sex.

- The hormone that is first associated with pregnancy is **human chorionic gonadotropin** (**HCG**). This is what is detected in your blood through a pregnancy test. In the first twelve weeks, the level of HCG rises dramatically, ensuring the safe implantation of the embryo and the growth of your placenta. Unfortunately, its main side effect is nausea. Not all women feel nauseous either in the first trimester or at any other time during pregnancy; however, those who do, really do. It goes without saying that the sexual impact of HCG as it relates to nausea is rather negative. When your tummy starts to churn, it's definitely difficult to get in the mood for sex.

So, ladies, as you navigate your pregnancy, keep in mind that these hormones are preparing your entire body to carry and deliver your baby. But they also have dramatic effects on your sexuality—some wildly delicious, others rather daunting.

Your Blood Is Pumping!

Ever since you found out you were pregnant, have you noticed a subtle swelling of your privates? What about sudden bouts of dizziness as you stand up too quickly or bend down to shave your legs? If you are fair skinned, have you noticed an increase in the size of the blood vessels just beneath the surface of your skin? Your body is producing up to 20 percent (or one liter) *more* blood—composed of plasma and red and white blood cells. Although this increase is gradual throughout your pregnancy, women do feel an immediate impact, especially in how they respond sexually. The additional blood and oxygen in your system enhance the sexual excitation and orgasms.

Specifically, the three most significant effects of this increase that relate to sexuality have to do with 1) the engorgement of tissue; 2) an increase in the intensity of orgasms; and 3) headaches. Clearly the first two side effects of this increase in blood benefit your sexual pleasure and functioning—who would turn down more sensation and pleasure? Unfortunately, headaches are not usually conducive to getting you in the mood for sex. But let's see how to make the most of your body's changes.

SWELLING PRIVATES AND NEW SENSITIVITIES

The engorgement of tissue means all tissues—from the lips on your face to the lips in your vagina. Not only do many men find this swelling a turn-on, many women experience an increase in sensation and arousal. Lena described the change this way: "I was just bigger down there—with more to play with and more for my husband to enjoy." The increase in blood flow generally leads to engorgement of both inner and outer labia and the clitoris, deepening their hue. The genitals may also become softer and swollen, as during arousal. Courtney told me that just walking down the street was arousing because of the friction that was created down there. "It was similar to that feeling just after having sex. Everything between my legs just tingled."

Most women I have talked to say the resulting sensitivity is a terrific turn-on. You tingle when he brushes against the back of your leg. Suddenly the crown of your head is alive with sensation. Parts of your body that never felt sexy before are getting you all hot and bothered. What is going on? According to Dr. Marc Ganem, whose book *La Sexualité du couple pendant la grossesse* is based on a study of more than six hundred couples during pregnancy, the increased blood flow leads to a shift and an expansion of pre-pregnancy erogenous zones for many women. So instead of thinking of your genitals and breasts as the only two zones of erotic pleasure, tap into other parts of your body that may now be energized by this increase in blood flow. Does the crown of your head feel more sensitive? Your lower back? Your feet? The inside of your arm, at the crux of your elbow? Dr. Ganem writes that some women report feeling aroused in so-called outlying areas such as the flanks, the hands, and the backs of the legs. In other words, your skin becomes more of a sensual playground, which is related to the profusion of new blood in your body. The possibilities are endless—if you stay open, focused, and willing to explore your body's new sensations.

ORGASM

Since orgasms are naturally powered by blood, some women who are highly charged to begin with experience more intense orgasms as their pregnancy progresses. "During my first trimester and throughout my pregnancy, it definitely took me longer to orgasm, but when I came, I came with a bang. It was a whole new feeling." That's the way Shannon described the new intensity of her orgasms once she was pregnant. Holly explained the change in her orgasm this way: "I was so engorged that my husband would barely lick me and I was brought to orgasm. Never mind that I began to masturbate more just to let off some steam—I finally understood the physical release that men always describe." Stephanie linked the increase in the intensity of her orgasm to the expansion of her uterus. As she said, "There was just so much more of me to get excited, and the result was this outrageously deep orgasm."

Some women said it took them longer to climax, but it was worth the wait: "They took longer to happen, but as intensity goes, they started from where my biggest nonpregnant orgasms ended and took off from there. Sometimes they took me out of my body, and other times it was like I felt them in places I hadn't expected—my toes, my tongue, my arms."

You may fall in either camp—you may orgasm more slowly or more quickly—but it seems more than likely that you will experience an increase in intensity. But you are certainly not going to find this level of intensity unless you try—as little Mikey used to say on the Life cereal commercials, "Try it, you'll like it."

Unfortunately, some women, for no clear physiological reason, have trouble orgasming while pregnant. If this is the case, try channeling your erotic energy into a more sensual connection with yourself and your partner. Massage, caresses, and kissing are a few of the things that can help you stay connected and experience pleasure—without the focus (or pressure) of sex and orgasm.

*C*an Having an Orgasm During the First Trimester Induce a Miscarriage?

The experts say *no*! Even if there is some cramping or spotting after sexual intercourse or masturbation, this does *not* increase the danger of losing your fetus. Here are the facts about miscarriage in the first trimester:

- About 85 percent of miscarriages occur in the first twelve weeks of pregnancy, according to *The Merck Manual of Diagnosis and Therapy: General Medicine.*
- Of that 85 percent, 80 percent of miscarriages are due to "chromosomal abnormality incompatible with life," according to Dr. Jules Black. This means that Mother Nature is taking its course and rejecting a nonviable

fetus. There is nothing a mother can or cannot do to prevent such an outcome.

- "Sexual activity has not been shown to contribute to miscarriage. This applies to intercourse in almost any position, to oral sex, and to masturbation," points out Dr. Henry M. Lerner.
- Specifically, there is no relation between orgasms and miscarriage. "An exception to this would be if, during the first four months of your pregnancy you were to have vaginal bleeding or spotting," writes Dr. Henry M. Lerner. See page 44 for more information.
- According to Dr. Marc Ganem, making love cannot be responsible for either the survival or the termination of the fetus's well-being, and any association of having sex and a miscarriage creates a "useless culpability."

For further information on the causes of miscarriage beyond chromosomal abnormalities, consult your ob-gyn or Dr. Henry M. Lerner's very extensive and complete book, *Miscarriage: Why It Happens and How Best to Reduce Your Risks— A Doctor's Guide*.

Those Bodacious Boobs

Women are often astounded by the changes in their breast size—even in these first three months. For many who have gone through life as an A or a B cup, bodaciousness in the breast department can add a whole new sense of sexiness. As Kristina, a thirty-five-year-old pregnant client, shared, "I want to make use of these incredible boobs. I know they won't be here long!" I know one woman who went from a B cup to a D cup during her first pregnancy, did not nurse, remained a slightly larger D throughout her second pregnancy, again not nursing, and still has her D size intact. She also swears a friend's tip to wear a bra at *all* times saved her from having *National Geographic* boobs. (See pages 200–201 for tips on how to maintain the shape, tone, and elasticity of your breasts once you deliver.)

Grant, the loving husband of Claire, said this about his wife's increase in breast size: "I like large breasts, and I happened to marry a woman who is very small chested—no big deal. But when she got pregnant, she went from a small B to a DD. Not only did I enjoy playing with her breasts, she could orgasm while I licked and sucked on her nipples—something she was never able to do before!"

Alas, not all women experience such a radical increase in the size of their breasts. As Marty said, "I've been a small B my entire life, and I was finally going to have a great chest and the titty fairy missed my house." Connie said she went up only a half size during pregnancy and then another half size once she delivered and began nursing. *C'est la vie.*

There is another breast factor to consider beyond any size issues: during the first trimester, this swelling of the breasts can lead to tenderness, tingling, or soreness in the breast or nipples. Some women enjoy this extra sensitivity, but others find such sensitivity bothersome and don't want anyone touching them. As Charles stated, "I was thrilled that Megan's breasts got bigger, but the sad part was I couldn't play with them—they were too sore."

You may also notice a darkening of the areola or an elevation of the glands around the nipple (they look like goose bumps). Marybeth told me that her "nipples got huge and dark with large bumps around the areola. It took a while for my partner to get used to the new look. Then, when he did, he loved sucking on them."

For most women neither the positive aspects nor the negatives of the new breasts will last forever. The too-sensitive-to-touch sensitivity for most women lasts until the fifth month. As Georgia stated, "By the time my breasts were no longer sensitive, poor Barry was so used to my leaping out of my skin with any touch, we had to relearn how to touch my breasts." And as I indicated above, once women deliver, they usually grow at least one more bra size—if they continue to nurse.

How to Make the Most of Your Fabulous New Figure

In your first trimester, as your breasts grow and your blood flow enlarges your lips—both sets!—consider enhancing your new curves:

- Indulge in a low-cut sweater or shirt to show off that cleavage.
- Now is the time to get some *Playboy* Bunny–style lingerie to accent those breasts, before your belly makes it impossible.
- Never had the nerve to wear a clinging halter dress? Try one on for size.
- Experiment with a pencil skirt. As your breasts and waistline grow, your hips and thighs will look in proportion to the rest of you, allowing you to look smashing in a slim-line skirt.

Eating for Two? The Way You Eat Can Affect the Way You Feel

Ladies, my sincerest advice to you is to be careful not to go hog wild with eating. As one wise mother of three said to me, "If you hear anyone tell you to go ahead and have that second or third slice of pizza or cake because you're eating for two, just remind them—yeah, me and six ounces!"

Some women lose weight at the beginning of their pregnancies, but most will retain their original weight or gain just two to four pounds during their first trimester. Why so little? you may ask. In many ways, the growing fetus inside of you acts like a parasite, taking what it needs from you. In this way, the food you eat does not nourish your baby, but you. The baby can take care of herself, taking as much nourishment from you as she needs and is available. Therefore your body needs only marginally more food than it did before pregnancy, but it needs nutrient-rich food, especially good protein. As Dr. Peter Nathanielsz points out, "During this time [when the organs are developing] the fetus takes everything from the mother, so you must be especially aware of good eating habits." However, he says plainly, "if you are eating well before pregnancy, there is no need to actively increase your calorie intake at the very beginning of pregnancy. You should gain only a pound a month in the first trimester. Gaining weight too quickly can lead to high blood pressure, which in turn can lead to preeclampsia, which can become a life-threatening condition." (Please see page 95 for more information on preeclampsia.)

THE BEST PRENATAL NUTRITION

During pregnancy it's more important than ever to eat a healthy balance of foods from all the different food groups. Dr. Nathanielsz recommends in his book *The Prenatal Prescription* that women use the USDA Food Guide Pyramid as a general guide to eating because it provides descriptions of the five essential groups. (I would be remiss if I didn't point out that many nutritionists today are questioning not only the makeup of the food pyramid but its ranking and portioning of the various food groups.) In my discussions with nutritionists, they emphasize that though we need to eat from all food categories, balance and moderation are necessary. Also key is careful selection of food. Here are some general recommendations for pregnant women:

- ➤ Rely most heavily on complex carbohydrates (such as whole grains).
- ➤ Watch your intake of starchy carbohydrates (white flour, rice, and pasta), and when you do eat such foods, combine them with protein to slow down their impact on your blood sugar.

- Eat as much as you want from the fruit and vegetable group, as they are both vital, nutrient-rich sources of vitamins and minerals.
- Include two or three servings of protein from the milk group and/or the meat and beans group; protein is essential for you and your baby.
- Watch your intake of the top group—fats, oils, and sugary foods such as junk food, baked goods, and candy. These fatty foods fill you up with little or no nutritional value.
- Avoid processed foods as much as possible. The preservatives, fat content, and low nutritional value make them empty calories.

A *Vegetarian Pregnancy**

You can be a vegetarian, stay healthy, and give your growing baby all the necessary nutrition during pregnancy. According to Heidi Murkoff, coauthor of the bestselling *What to Expect When You're Expecting*, vegetarians need to pay special attention to these dietary requirements:

- **Protein**—you can get your recommended sixty grams of protein from legumes, nuts, whole grains, and meat substitutes such as veggie burgers.
- **Calcium**—if you don't eat dairy, get your calcium from tofu, green leafy vegetables, beans, broccoli, and calcium-fortified soy milk or orange juice.
- **Vitamin B$_{12}$**—it is usually included in your prenatal vitamin, but make sure.
- **Vitamin D**—milk and soy milk are fortified with this important vitamin.

*as reported in *Healthy Pregnancy*, Spring/Summer 2004.

Ladies, the most important factor to keep in mind in terms of eating and gaining weight is to stay connected to your body. Many women still like to think of pregnancy as a time to eat with abandon. They not only increase their portion sizes, but they begin to eat more fattening, sugary, or starchy foods—all of which not only have negative health consequences but also increase your weight gain. This increase in weight gain is onerous: after you deliver you will have that much more weight to lose. Why take the risk? Also, gaining too much weight during pregnancy can have negative consequences for how you experience yourself. So my advice is to eat in moderation, take care of yourself, and listen to your own body for what it needs.

But that doesn't mean depriving yourself of treats or cravings. Carrie told me that she gave herself a reward each day—a chocolate chip cookie, some ice cream. "I looked forward to that treat every day. I ended up gaining forty pounds—about ten more than I had wanted to. But in the end, I accepted that that was the way I handled the situation. But it's the ten pounds I am still trying to lose five months later!" Marie said that during her second pregnancy, she paid less attention to what she was eating and simply ate in a balanced way. "Some people might say I broke all the rules: I drank one cup of coffee each morning, I ate some sushi that I knew was absolutely fresh and high quality, and I had a bowl of ice cream three or four nights a week. There are so many rules—no deli meats, no caffeine, no blue cheese—I was going crazy. But when you really do the research, the risk of infection is minimal—doctors just need to be conservative. And guess what, I not only gained less weight than I did with my first baby, my second baby arrived in perfect health and weighing eight pounds three ounces!" You may not want to be as adventurous or cavalier as Marie, but take her attitude to heart and be easy on yourself.

That said, I do want to underscore the importance of moderation and balance. As modern women, we all know that how we feel externally about ourselves is very much related to how we feel internally about ourselves. If we are feeling unappealing externally, we often feel insecure internally, and vice versa. The tension of this internal-external pull is even more intense during pregnancy, when women are forced to deal with a pretty drastic change in self-image. Your mirror does not lie: you are indeed getting bigger. And when we deal with this issue, some women immediately withdraw—especially sexually. This potential for withdrawal, of course, is where my concern lies. I've seen long-term couples begin to come apart and relationships unravel because the woman who has gained so much weight has much more of a tendency to withdraw from her partner, leaving not only him stranded but also the relationship.

Weight Gain at a Glance— Keeping It in Perspective

There is no avoiding the fact that you will gain weight during your pregnancy. After all, there is a whole new person growing inside of you. And while there is no ideal weight gain (because of variations in body type, metabolism, pre-pregnancy weight, the size of your baby, and your nutrition), most women gain twenty-five to forty pounds over the course of their pregnancies. Be careful not to get obsessed with how much or little you seem to be gaining. There is a lot of variation among women, with some women gaining as much as sixty pounds per pregnancy and other women gaining under twenty-five pounds.

The Challenges of the First Trimester: Fatigue, Nausea, and Other Concerns

FATIGUE: NOT TONIGHT, HONEY, I'M TOO TIRED

One of the most common complaints I hear from my newly pregnant clients is exhaustion. As you have just seen, your body is going through unprecedented physical adjustments, and you will probably feel these effects as waves of fatigue. One woman told me about her pregnant sister who actually fell asleep on the train on the commute home and woke up an hour and a half away from her train stop. But don't despair, ladies, this bone-weary tiredness will pass after the first three months, when the biggest construction process of pregnancy is established. By this time, the fetus and the placenta are firmly in place and growing. As you will see in the second trimester, from this point on the growth the fetus undergoes is more of an expansion. So keep in mind the first trimester motto: this too shall pass.

The excitement of knowing you and your mate have created a human being that is steadily flourishing inside can give you renewed energy. But all some women seem to long for is sleep, sleep, and more sleep. It is important to honor how you feel. Jesse said this about fatigue and sex: "I was working half days, and when I walked in the door at three P.M., all I wanted to do was crawl into bed for the night. I would think, 'How am I going to stay awake until Mark gets home at six?' Then I got in the habit of taking quick power naps. Sometimes I didn't even sleep, but allowing myself twenty or thirty minutes to lie there with my eyes closed did the trick. I started to feel my whole attitude shift, and I realized that one of the biggest factors of my fatigue was trying to fight it. Once I let myself off the hook and accepted that I needed a nap, I felt better for the rest of the day. Then when Mark and I got into bed, I didn't feel the need to collapse and turn away from him."

Jesse brings up an important point. The fatigue is not only physical; it's emotional. When women deny their exhaustion or feel as if they shouldn't feel exhausted, then they usually make matters worse. You need to respect how your body is feeling. Your fatigue is a sign that your body is working overtime to build and sustain life, and that you need to rest. On the other hand, in interviewing hundreds of women, it became clear that many women stay away from sex during the first trimester because they interpret their body's fatigue as a warning signal to stop doing the things they love to do, including having sex. Rest when you need to, but don't stop what you're doing—unless you want to. Your fatigue may interfere nicely with your motivation to clean out your garage or do a half hour on a Spin bike, but don't deny yourself pleasure completely. If your physician or medical professional has told you that you are having a normal pregnancy and you are otherwise in good health, then continue what you've been doing—working, having fun, exercising, and yes, having sex.

MORNING SICKNESS AND NAUSEA

If you are one of the walking wounded, frequently finding yourself doubled over in discomfort from nausea and morning sickness, keep in mind that relief is more than likely on its way. In the vast majority of cases, women say their nausea subsides between the twelfth and the fourteenth week. As Dr. Gil Mileikowsky stated, the true pregnancy hormone is human chorionic gonadotropin (HCG), whose source is the developing fetal placenta. Production begins very early in pregnancy, almost certainly by the day of implantation. Thereafter, HCG levels in maternal plasma and urine rise very rapidly. With a sensitive test, it can be detected in maternal plasma or urine by eight or nine days after ovulation.

I daresay, it may be a bit difficult to feel excited about or interested in sex when you are feeling nauseous, but before you close the door on your spouse, you need to keep in mind one simple idea: sexual desire and orgasm can help counteract or lessen your morning sickness. While my support for this is mostly anecdotal, I have been told by a number of women that after sex, their nausea abated. "There's no doubt about it: having sex made my nausea disappear. The hard part was getting myself to start," says Val, twenty-eight. Some scientific findings point to a possible biological explanation: the increase in oxygen circulation during sex may help mediate the nausea in a similar way that increasing oxygen inhalation reduces the ill side effects of too much alcohol. Oxygen is a vasoconstrictor that counteracts the vasodilation impact of alcohol. At the very least, this potential nausea remedy is worth a try, isn't it? It certainly has to be more fun than eating another sleeve of saltines.

Morning Sickness— What's Going On?

Several facts about your nausea and morning sickness:

- According to Dr. Jules Black, your nausea is a result of how the section of your brain called the hypothalamus mediates (interprets) the rapidly increasing HCG during your early weeks of pregnancy.
- One of the reasons for the body's intense reaction to this rise in HCG is how quickly it increases in concentration, doubling in 1.4 to 2.0 days. These levels continue to increase, peaking at about sixty to seventy days. Thereafter, the concentration declines slowly until a low point is reached at about 100 to 130 days (Williams Obstetrics 21st edition, p. 27).
- Morning sickness can occur any time of day, but most often it starts early, as that is when the HCG levels are highest in your body, and the nausea abates as you become more active throughout the day.
- There is no known cure, though a medication called Bendectin (Debendox) that did work was pulled from the market in 1983 due to the legal costs associated with the defense of unproved allegations of congenital anomalies—even though the company won all cases that went to court.

Here are some standard suggestions for combating morning sickness and nausea:

- Eat frequently but keep your portions small. Carry snack food (saltines, trail mix, nuts) at all times. Carbohydrates and proteins are your allies.
- Avoid spicy, heavy foods with strong odors: for once, bland is grand!
- Keep hydrated. Water is best. Sugary sodas or drinks with artificial sweeteners are not good for you, nor is caffeine, as they only dehydrate you. You may also find the taste of them off-putting.
- Try using lemon peels steeped in hot water as a soothing drink.
- One cure suggested by a Jewish grandmother was to sniff orange peels—the scent is supposed to help abate nausea.
- A recent Australian study by Caroline Smith published by the American College of Obstetricians and Gynecologists said that "ginger was equivalent to vitamin B_6 in reducing nausea, retching, and vomiting."
- Stay away from tobacco smoke (a wise idea even if you feel great).
- Take it easy: get up slowly, try not to rush, and indulge yourself in sensuous and comforting activities like a gentle massage. You may also enjoy a chair massage if lowering your head is too much.

To be honest, there are those women for whom nothing seemed to work. As Tracy, the mother of three boys, including one pair of twins, pointed out, "Throughout both of my pregnancies, I was sick as a dog for nine months. Nothing seemed to help—not exercise, not crackers, nothing. The doctor said I was just very sensitive. The only thing that made me feel any better was my doctor suggesting that my nausea might be a way my body was protecting the babies." Indeed, mothers of multiples often experience more nausea, as their HCG levels are even higher.

And remember: if you're really suffering, no one expects you to be a hero. Submitting to sex just to please your partner is never a good idea. But a nice cuddle can work wonders. Feeling your warm skin against your partner's body might be just the pick-me-up you could use. (Some women feel constantly chilled during early pregnancy; stroking or cuddling can help with that, too.)

Some Risks and Warnings to Consider

While most women experience no physiological limitations to having sex during their first trimester, there are some conditions that preclude sex, especially intercourse, during this time. Consider the following list. Much of this information has been gathered from Dr. Glade B. Curtis's very informative book *Your Pregnancy Week by Week* and substantiated by my panel of experts. If you experience any of these symptoms, it would be wise to consult your health care professional to make sure it is safe for you to be active sexually. Also, you may want to be proactive and ask your health care provider if you might be at risk for any of these conditions.

SPOTTING—WHAT IT CAN MEAN

Many women notice spotting (small amounts of blood) during pregnancy. Up to 30 percent of women experience some bleeding or cramping at least once during the first twenty weeks of pregnancy, and this is perfectly normal. However, if bleeding becomes excessive, then you should consult your physician and stop having sexual intercourse.

COULD YOU STILL BE GETTING YOUR PERIOD?

You may not even know you're pregnant at first, especially if you are experiencing consistent bleeding or spotting in your first trimester. This happened to a friend of mine, who assumed—as most of us would—that it was a continuation of her menses. But this is where pregnant women are thrown a curveball. There are two possible reasons for such bleeding, neither of which is a cause for concern. First, normal implantation of the fertilized egg in the uterine wall might cause light bleeding. Second, until the growing embryo and placenta occupy the entire uterine chamber, there may be a very light bleed (called decidual bleed) that feels like a period because it comes at the normal monthly time. Such bleeding is usually less than a typical period, as there is less of an area from which to bleed. After about twelve or thirteen weeks, when the fetus occupies the entire uterus, the endometrium is obliterated, and this bleeding will stop.

So rest assured you do indeed know your body. You are not nuts; you just didn't know this little known piece of information. My friend's periods were only one or two days in duration, so she was blindsided last year when she found out she was four months pregnant.

BLEEDING AFTER INTERCOURSE

During pregnancy, the mouth of your uterus becomes crisscrossed with countless new blood vessels to accommodate that extra blood flow, and the tissue of the cervix and the vagina can sometimes suffer from abrasions during intercourse, or deep penetration. Don't assume that such bleeding means your baby has been harmed, and don't freak out. One husband did just that. Martha recalled, "One time after sex, my husband pulled out of me looking like he'd been shot in the penis. Once he figured out he was fine, he stopped freaking out . . . until he realized it was me! Of course, there was nothing wrong—my cervix was just supersensitive."

It is important to know that fetal blood does *not* mix with your blood, so this is about your system, not the baby's. One woman reported that during sex, the end of her husband's penis bumped the mouth of her cervix. Some of the capillaries burst, causing bleeding. Dr. Black adds that since during pregnancy, the cervix presents in a more open position, it exposes more of the fragile columnar cells, which are vulnerable to bleeding. This kind of bleeding is not dangerous, unless it continues well after sex. Remember, if you bleed consistently or in large amounts, always notify your physician.

EXCESSIVE BLEEDING

Certainly, there are times when excessive blood can be a warning sign of a condition known as placenta previa, which occurs when the placenta is attached very low in the uterus, either covering or very close to the cervix. According to standard reports, placenta previa is rather rare, occurring in one out of every 170 pregnancies. Its most characteristic symptom is painless bleeding without uterine contractions. Although some research indicates that spontaneous miscarriages can occur because of placenta previa, ultrasound technology can identify the problem, though it is often hard to diagnose until the second trimester. Since the placenta spans the cervix, which has a canal, there are some blood vessels of the placenta spanning the opening as well. Therefore, it is best for women with placenta previa to abstain from vaginal intercourse. However, you do have other options, which you will find in the next chapter.

When Are You at Risk for Placenta Previa?

If you have had previous cesareans or many pregnancies or are an older mom and experience heavy bleeding during non-pregnant sex, make sure to check with your doctor.

CRAMPING

In six weeks your uterus has grown from the size of a fist to that of a grapefruit. As it grows and your varicosity increases, you may feel cramping or even pain in your lower abdomen, or tightening or contractions of the uterus. This is not a miscarriage; in fact, it can occur during and after orgasm. It's also very common and harmless during a normal low-risk pregnancy. The cause can be physical (normal venous congestion of the pelvic area and sexual organs) or even psychological (fear of hurting the baby). However, please note that a severe or lengthy bout of cramping or bleeding—especially if not associated with sex or orgasm—warrants an immediate call to your doctor.

BEWARE OF TOXINS DURING THE FIRST TRIMESTER

During the first six weeks after conception (or eight weeks from your last menstrual period), organogenesis takes place: this is when the fetus's organs, heart, limbs, gonads, eyes, and central nervous system are formed. This is the most crucial period for adverse drug and substance impact on the fetus; it starts at twenty days after conception and continues through the fifty-fifth day. So be most careful of ingesting or being exposed to toxins such as:

- drugs or alcohol;
- high amounts of artificial sweeteners, such as saccharin and aspartame;
- household cleaners that contain ammonia and other toxic ingredients (it's best to use rubber/latex gloves when handling such products);
- strong chemicals used in nail salons, including nail polish remover and quick dry sprays (and make sure your nail salon is well ventilated).

Hair Dye: To Stop or Not

Many women are loath to stop coloring their hair while pregnant. And while the conservative party line of most physicians is to stop using any dye while pregnant because of the slight risk of the dye penetrating the mother's skin and then the placenta, I consulted Dr. Jules Black, who assured me that after forty years as an ob-gyn he has never witnessed a problem related to hair dye. By *dye* I mean any semipermanent or permanent coloring product—either store-bought or used in a salon. The general concern of American physicians is that the chemicals in hair dye might penetrate the skin of the scalp and adversely affect your baby. This has never been proved to be true. Dr. Black adds, "Experience among my colleagues has shown that in less litigious but civilized societies overseas, there is no danger to the fetus of standard hairdressing procedures." If, however, you are still concerned that the chemicals used in hair dye may be absorbed into your blood and thereby impact your growing baby, try such options as highlights (the foils don't touch the scalp) or henna, which is a vegetable-based product containing no man-made chemicals.

Throughout your first trimester, your body is undergoing stress as it shifts into maternal mode. Be patient, be kind—with yourself, that is. If you feel like taking the plunge into full Hot Mama status, then do so. If you're still warming up to the suggestions of how to stay in touch with your man sexually and sensually, then take your time. But do try to take care of yourself, and honor your body and mind as they begin to transform right before your very eyes.

In the next chapter I will tease you a bit more into what's waiting for you as a Hot Mama. You will find great tips on how to have pleasurable sex—despite your fatigue and tender breasts. You will also find some other options that may just tickle your fancy. And on we go!

3

Sex and Saltines

Positions and Tips for the First Trimester

W OMEN FALL INTO SEVERAL CAMPS when it comes to their relationship to sex during their first three months of pregnancy.
Some women crave the normalcy of intimacy at a time when everything seems to be changing, for others it is not even on the radar, while
others still just want to get right down to it—thanks to Mother Nature's raging hormones at their best. Other women have described
their desire for sexual pleasure as a need to stay as close to their men as
possible. As Jackie explained, "Maybe I was sort of freaking out in my
own way—I just wanted to be with him at all times, and that meant
sexually as well."

But there are plenty of pregnant women who find it a challenge to
stay in or get into the groove for sex. As any pregnant woman who has
suffered from nausea or tender breasts will tell you, this time period is
about changing touch and adjusting position to not aggravate either.

The good news is that from a physiological standpoint, you have
plenty of choices for intercourse and manual, oral, and anal sex. If you
like to play with toys, then go ahead and enjoy yourselves. For the first
three months, most women's bodies do not present any restrictions on
any sexual activity (within their own comfort zone), so you need not
give up your favorite and best positions.

If, however, you are one of those women for whom breast tenderness and nausea get in the way of fully opening yourself sexually, there

are simple ways to adjust parts of your intimate connections. So whether you choose the bedroom, the living room, or the backyard for your activities, I have incorporated the suggestions from the surveyed couples as to what worked best for them.

Woman on Top

These positions are likely going to be some of your best options throughout your pregnancy, but never more so than during the first three months, when your body has not begun outwardly changing. The beauty of these moves is that the woman on top is in charge of the amount of motion and the intensity and depth of penetration by her partner. Some women say they prefer being more upright to avoid triggering nausea. Other women focus on the positions that allow for more subdued motion. Women who want to cover their bases, so to speak, may enjoy sitting in a chair, a specific pose that some couples now refer to as the Sex Chair position. In this position, you are in control of both important factors.

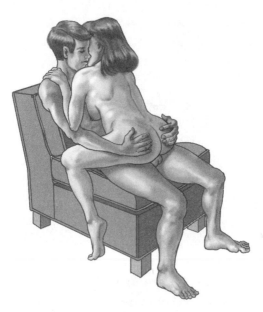

Fig. 1

Should you be one of the lucky ladies who do not experience morning sickness, you may find there is little to no change in your intimate activities aside from your extra-sensitive breasts. Figure 2 showcases a lady who is able to do as she pleases and establish the clitoral connection that works best for her.

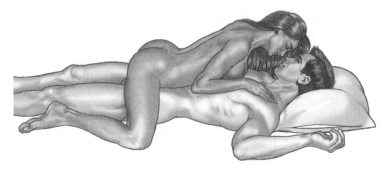

Fig. 2

In figure 3 the lady is astride her man facing away from him. Depending on her preference, she is able to stimulate with his shaft, her fingers, or a toy both her clitoral area and, depending on her angle, the front vaginal wall for better G spot sensation.

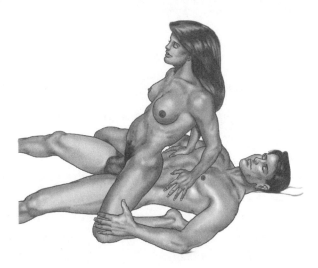

Fig. 3

Rear Entry (aka Doggie Style)

Couples who enjoy Man from Behind (aka Rear Entry or Doggie Style) positions are likely to find the purest form of this position with the lady on all fours (as in figure 4) the best, as it avoids the lady's leaning on anything and putting pressure on her breasts or abdomen. In figure 4 we see a woman who prefers support under her tummy.

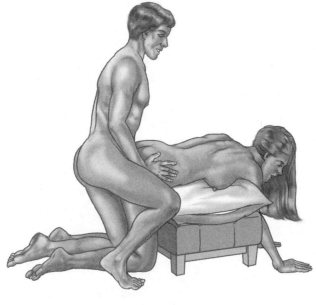

Fig. 4

Oral Pleasures

Oral aficionados are going to be in their element, as the increased genital sensitivity (thanks to your pumped-up hormones) will enhance this form of pleasure. Also, when a lady is orally stimulating a man, she may find that he tastes more metallic than before, which is probably due to the woman's increased gum sensitivity. The small amount of blood excreted may taste metallic.

The Tahitian Method, presented by Dr. Patti Britton, is a worldwide hit in my Sexuality Seminars. The beauty of this method, as seen in figure 5, is that a partner can create intense oral stimulation for a woman while getting immediate feedback from her that they are in the right place. You can also use this method to add a new angle for both of you.

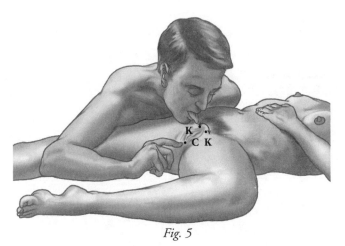

Fig. 5

For ease of explanation, locate the *k* and *c* points on the diagram. Then follow the directions below:

- The man lies perpendicular to the woman.
- The woman's only responsibility is to receive sensation.
- The partner uses a back-and-forth tongue stroke over the hood of the clitoris. Men who have practiced this technique have said that when the woman is aroused, they can feel two small bumps on either side of the clitoral hood that feel like half grains of rice. These are the *k* points.
- The *c* point is where the man gets immediate feedback from the woman that he is in the right place. The man places his middle finger on her perineum, the *c* point, which is the area between the vagina and the anus. The partner should make sure his nails are short so the woman can feel only his finger pad, not his nail. The reason he will get immediate feedback is that when he is stroking in the correct place, the woman will experience involuntary pre-orgasmic contractions in this area. By reading her body, he will

be able to maintain correct tongue placement without wondering, "Am I there? Where is there? Have I moved from there?"

- The finger on the *c* point does not move or pulse. It needs to remain nonmoving to feel the subtlety of the preorgasmic contractions and to not distract the woman by creating sensation in an area other than the one he wants attention paid to.
- Once the man has started, he shouldn't stop. He should continue past the woman's initial orgasmic response, as often this stimulation is the most intense and satisfying portion of the orgasm.
- Some couples have added a position adjustment: the woman curls her legs up to her chest, and the man uses his arm to keep them pushed back and stabilized. In this way, the woman is very widely spread open and can receive even more intense stimulation.

Using Support Devices to Enhance Pleasure

As with all things during your pregnancy, chances are creativity will become your middle name. Anyone who has read any of my other books knows that I feel pillows are one of your best sex toys. During this time I also recommend a line of props from OneUp Innovations LLC called Liberator® Shapes, described below (for more information on the products, go to *www.tryliberator.com* or call the toll-free number 866/542-7283). These four innovative shapes can assist in your activities while you are trying to get pregnant and are a boon to maintaining positions during and after pregnancy. Field researchers, both pregnant and nonpregnant, have found two of the Liberator® Shapes—the Liberator® Wedge and the Liberator® Ramp—and their possible combinations—to be their favorite shapes.

Erika reported, "We first heard about these pillows as products that could be used to help you get pregnant. We have always used pillows when we have sex, so these seemed like a great idea for pregnancy. What we didn't expect was they could be used throughout and afterward for equally good results. They were a godsend as I got bigger because our regular pillows just weren't enough. Depending on our mood, usually mine, we were able to keep having sex up until the day before Josh was born."

Georgia shared, "The full-length body pillows were great for getting and keeping both of us in positions when I was pregnant. I get big really fast, so my body pillow was my new best friend, and my husband loved being 'l'artiste' by sculpting new shapes with it to support me while we made love."

THE LIBERATOR® RAMP AND WEDGE

There is an ergonomically sound design idea behind the Liberator® Ramp (24"–30" W x 34"–36" L x 12"–14" H) and the Liberator® Wedge (24"–30" W x 14" x 7" H). They both use long, gentle sloping foam support shapes that enable both partners to relax more into the sensations because they are not distracted by having to maintain balance or getting tired while doing so. The Liberator® Shapes have a velvety soft blue cover that keeps you in place so you can concentrate on your pleasure and not worry about slipping. The soft cover can be zippered off for easy laundering.

Figure 6 shows but one of the rear entry position possibilities when combining the two shapes, whether on the bed or the floor—only your imagination limits any placement option.

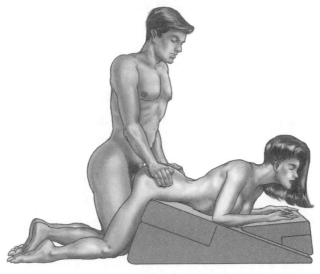

Fig. 6

The beauty of these two items is in their ergonomic design and their ability to be used together to expand your position options, as shown in figures 7 and 8. However, supportive devices work whether you choose a prefabricated technology such as the Liberator® Shapes or use your own foam shape or pillows.

Figure 7 shows a male superior position using the smaller Liberator® Wedge. Her legs are wrapped above his back to help maintain the closeness through the hip pelvic area, and her delicate stomach will have less jostling than a flat-on-the-bed position might cause. He is able to thrust more easily because his knees have the side of the Liberator® Wedge to brace against, again lessening the jostling of his partner.

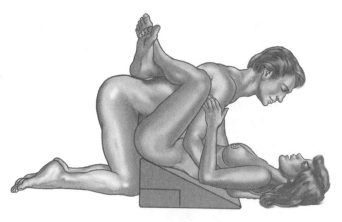

Fig. 7

Figure 8 shows the Liberator® Ramp in use with the gentleman in a standing or kneeling position. Because he doesn't have to use his inner thigh strength to maintain his position, as he would in a standard male superior position, he will experience less fatigue. At the same time, the lady can relax into the sensations, as there is no effort on her part to maintain position. The man is also able to sustain firm penetration because gravity keeps their groins close without any weight being put on the woman. She can use the strength of her legs on his shoulders to adjust to her preferred angle, and he can use his upper-body strength—his arms hold the front of her thighs to establish a more finessed thrusting. And depending on her preference, she can determine the depth of penetration by varying her hip angle and/or varying how widely she spreads her legs.

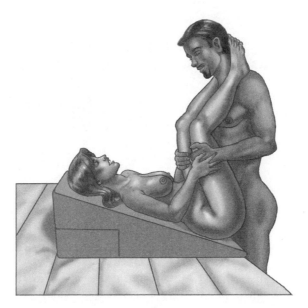

Fig. 8

Tips for Sensual Challenges of the First Trimester

NAUSEA AND EXHAUSTION

Should you experience nausea and exhaustion, keep in mind that less is more in the motion department, and use any position that invloves little to no pressure on your abdomen. This is the time that spooning sex takes the lead, as seen in figure 9, or the slow full-body contact of the woman seated on her man, as previously depicted in figure 1, in which she can also use the strength of her legs to adjust herself easily.

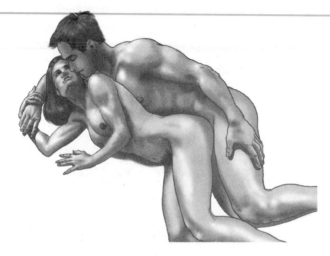

Fig. 9

Sensitive and Tender Breasts

Even if you adored breast stimulation pre-pregnancy (and as you may know, some women actually experience orgasms through such stimulation), you may find your growing orbs too tender for any play now. As one woman described her sensitivity, "Imagine your worst sunburn and how anything touching your skin—be it the air, water, sheets—feels *too* painful."

To put you more in control of the situation, consider investing in some great comfortable lingerie. Indeed, your sports bras may take on a new seduction function. As Marty shared with me, "I found the only thing that made my breasts even bearable was wearing a firm-fitting sports bra. By the end I had one in every color, and post-pregnancy they have become a part of our sex life. My husband especially likes the 'front-end loaders,' as he calls them, the front zipper style." Figure 10 illustrates the lingerie idea to keep her sensitive breasts protected. As you can see, the couple is still deeply connected, while avoiding putting pressure on her abdomen and breasts by using an angled position.

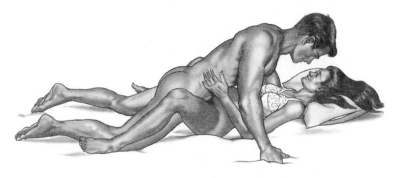

Fig. 10

Of course, do not limit yourselves to the positions I've described here—the world is your oyster. Many couples find great enjoyment in oral, manual, and anal play. As you will see in the next chapter, the impediments of fatigue and nausea often give way to luscious sex in the second trimester. As one husband of three children said, "The way my wife was during her pregnancies makes men pray that the nine months could last nine years."

The Second Trimester

4

Kindling the Fire Within and Revving Up Your Evolving Relationship

A s they stride into the second trimester, most women feel an enormous sense of relief: their nausea has faded or decreased, their fog of fatigue has begun to lift, and the mood and energy swings associated with hormonal changes have lessened or ceased. Marie told me something that was echoed by hundreds of women I spoke with about the second trimester: "I felt like myself again after three months of hell!"

Welcome back.

For many couples, once they reach twelve weeks, they experience a shift in the realness of the pregnancy, making it nearly impossible for pregnancy to be anything but a concrete reality. You have had three months to get your heads around the idea that you will soon have a baby; you are gratefully past the worrying stage; you have gone public with your news; and your physical manifestations are becoming more apparent on a daily basis. At this time, the major physical changes—the growing roundness of your tummy, the larger breasts, the new shadows on your skin—are matched step by step with major psychological changes. For some couples the psychological changes are hugely aphrodisiac in their impact. As Mark explained, "We went from not knowing how to have sex because everything hurt or having her be so sick during the first trimester to a whole new level of sex during the second trimester. I felt this surge of confidence that came from knowing it was me that got her pregnant, and she noticed it. Our lovemaking just went to another level."

Others experienced a more subtle psychological shift—they moved from a state of excitement and/or anxiety to a wonderful calmness. Kathryn said this to me: "We just both calmed down and stopped worrying. I was feeling so much better, and Tom was so relieved that everything was OK with the baby. We didn't even have to think about sex—we just had it, and lots of it, like we were floating along down a slow, easy river of sex." Their desire for each other had become the seduction. Other couples described this shift as more dramatic and thrilling, as they suddenly felt revved up sexually. Hillary explained the change this way: "It was like we were new lovers again. And I felt more, tingled more."

As you contemplate what to do with your renewed energy, I want you to remember that promise you made to yourself to stay connected to the reason you are pregnant in the first place: your sexual relationship with your man. More than anything else, women have remarked upon this transition from first to second trimester as a time when they felt a renewed connection to their partners. And what could be more satisfying than experiencing this bond sexually? So hang on for dear life. These next three months could be the most exhilarating of your pregnancy as your stomach swells and your vitality returns. But before we get into your body and its changes, and look at the sexual tips and positions that work for you at this stage, let's take a look at how your attitude can help kindle the fire within you and rev up your relationship.

Sensual Spring

One of the first ways women experience this transition from first to second trimester is in a dramatic awakening of their senses: their senses of smell, sight, taste, touch, and hearing often become intensely and newly heightened. As Amy, thirty-seven, shared with me, "Somewhere around week thirteen, it was like a whole new world came to life. Everything started tasting better, colors were brighter, and any touch to my skin felt *fabulous!*" Andrea, thirty-five, said this: "Suddenly in week fourteen, food never tasted so good. Nothing was more yummy than veggie pad thai with its many layers of spicy, peanut-buttery sweetness. Can't you tell it is a fond memory?!" Amy and Andrea are not alone.

Hundreds of women reported the same or similar experiences. This is what they said:

- Food tastes better.
- Skin sensors come alive.
- Particular scents become titillating.
- They felt a springlike reaction to the world around them. They came alive with the sensation of a breeze across the face or arm, the primal satisfaction in watching leaves turn, watching a baby with his mother, or feeling the cool sand beneath their feet on a hot summer day.
- Listening to music became a more multidimensional experience. Susan said, "I wasn't passively listening to my favorite CDs. I could actually feel myself open up and relax."

Such vivid responses to the sensual world made the women revel that much more in the natural beauty of their pregnancy. Claire described to me a sensation she had one day walking home. She had to stop—the air seemed sweeter, the birds seemed to sing more beautifully—she had such an inner sense of calm and peace. This integration of the senses not only helped the women feel connected to themselves, their bodies, and their growing babies inside the womb, it also helped them feel connected to a universal sense of life—an awareness that brought them closer to an ecstatic state. So give yourself the chance to experience an extension of the miracle growing inside of you by nurturing this renewed sensuality—even if it's the dead of winter!

Again, in pregnancy, it's easy to give in to the banality of tiredness. Instead of celebrating the wondrous growth happening within them, some women opt to withdraw, shut down, and turn off their awareness of the sensual world. May I make a suggestion? Keep in mind that at no time in your life will you ever be so intuitively connected to your environment. It is your choice (as with all life events) to revel in and enjoy the moment or wish it to pass quietly and quickly. This is about choosing an attitude of seeing the bottle either half full or half empty. As you contemplate your choice, here are some suggestions for eliciting the sensual spring inside and outside of you:

- Sink into a warm (not hot) bath.
- Share a gentle massage with your partner, using lightly scented oils on your feet, hands, and tummy.
- Wear silky, soft fabrics that feel delicious against your skin—cashmere is particularly comforting.
- Visit a playground nearby in the afternoon and listen to the sweet voices of children playing.
- Weather permitting, take a stroll through a park, at the seaside, or in a nature preserve.
- Experiment with foods that are equally flavorful and light. (Many women complain that heavy foods, rich in oil or fat, trigger nausea.) Such ethnic cuisines as Thai, Vietnamese, Mediterranean, and Japanese use wonderful aromatic spices but don't have the density of heavier foods.
- Go to a candle store and spend some time finding a scented candle that appeals to you. You may discover that scents you used to prefer no longer appeal, or that you like some that you hadn't liked before. Women have told me that they prefer lighter, more floral scents, as opposed to heavier, spicier scents. Indeed, some women who want to initiate labor (at the end of their third trimester) use lemon oil in a water diffuser.
- Get a prenatal massage.
- Treat yourself to a facial and a relaxing neck and shoulder massage.
- Go to a concert with your lover.

Sensual Sensitivity

There are many wonderful ways to tickle the olfactory sense of a pregnant lady. Go ahead, take the time right now to quite literally stop and smell the . . .

- freshly baked cookies (Jamie, thirty-one, told me she used to stand outside the bakery near her apartment for ten minutes every morning on her way to work inhaling the delicious aroma. Of course, she always had to sample the wares, as well.)
- orange or lemon peels (help to alleviate nausea)
- baby powder (a scent of good things to come)
- first whiff of a newly opened box of chocolates
- sea air (There's something very earthy and warm about the salty, summery air at the beach.)
- freshly ground coffee (Some revel in the dark richness of it.)
- inky smell of the morning newspaper
- clean laundry

However, I would be remiss if I did not also point out that some women's new sensual sensitivity did have some drawbacks. One woman said that she would almost gag around perfume—"especially cheap perfume. One whiff and I wanted to barf." Another woman said that she found she couldn't be near the kitchen at dinner time (her husband cooked most nights—how lucky is she!) because the smell of raw meat sent her flying into the bathroom. Still another woman said that when she prepared chicken nuggets for her two-and-a-half-year-old, she could barely keep from dry heaving. My best advice? Avoid such strong odors at all costs.

TASTE BUD FEVER

Women have also reported that their taste buds change during pregnancy. Molly, a lifelong vegetarian, wanted only steak. Carly said she rarely ate vegetables before she was pregnant, but had to have sautéed spinach every day once she was pregnant. Both these foods—spinach and red meat—are high in iron, and both women reported being slightly anemic during pregnancy. So pay attention to your cravings and appreciate your new taste buds. Here is a sampling of favorite delectables during pregnancy:

- lemonade
- peanut butter—especially with a crunchy, crisp apple
- pickles (yes, really)
- apples, watermelon, and grapefruit
- anything tomato—sauce on spaghetti, salsa with tortilla chips, ketchup on a burger (if you're still eating meat)
- sour cream on anything
- red meat (One long-time vegetarian suddenly had to have a meatball sub every day for lunch.)
- white ice cream (This usually means vanilla. As one woman pointed out to me, "Anything else was too rich, but the creamy, velvet taste of vanilla was a narcotic for me.")

Odd Cravings

One woman said to her doctor, "I have the most disgusting craving for tabouli, and I hate tabouli. What is this all about?" The doctor responded, "Well, in your case it seems baby knows best. Your blood work shows that you have very low iron. Tabouli has a parsley base and is very iron rich."

Keeping Your Man Close

Just because you are feeling more energetic and comfortable with your pregnancy doesn't mean that your other half is not busy having all sorts of reactions to you and your pregnancy. I have found in talking to many men that it is during the second trimester that the reality of a baby on its way really hits them. Obviously, there are many reasons for wanting to keep your man close to you throughout your pregnancy, not the least of which is for your mental and emotional sanity. But it's also important to include him in your experience as much as possible and honor and respect his feelings, which may range from outright fear to nervousness to excitement to repulsion. Indeed, "men can have very complex feelings about what happens to their wives during pregnancy, but they often don't share them," says Greg Bishop, chairman of New Fathers Foundation, a nonprofit organization for first-time fathers in Irvine, California. And while most men report being very turned on by their pregnant wives, a small minority were hesitant to embrace their wives' swelling state. "I think all pregnant women look really cool," said one man. "The way they go through all sorts of wonderful transformations, it's almost like watching a construction project." Another man said, "We love swollen bellies." And still another man said, "There's nothing more beautiful than a woman carrying a child."

Some men experience their partners' pregnancy so intensely that they develop what is called Couvade syndrome, or a "sympathetic pregnancy." Armin Brott in his book *The Expectant Father: Facts, Tips, and Advice for Dads-to-Be* cites a study showing that almost 90 percent of expectant fathers experience Couvade syndrome at some point during their partners' pregnancy. This may explain why your man suddenly gains weight, experiences nausea, and has mood swings and food cravings!

Ladies, many men suddenly become shy around their pregnant wives. Some men have told me that they are afraid they will hurt the baby. Others have said they just become almost intimidated by the breadth of physical changes their ladies' bodies undergo. Please know that it is not weird or unusual for men to have this kind of reaction. As

David explained to me, "I felt like I was on the outside looking in, and I had no idea how to connect with her body anymore. I wanted to touch her, but at first I felt like a klutz—as if I should know and didn't."

Men also worry that they will not find their partners attractive—both during pregnancy and after. As Jack articulated, "The changes were so intense, it was like I couldn't keep up. All I kept thinking about was how her pregnancy was going to affect me, and—I know this sounds selfish—I worried that I was no longer going to be attracted to her." This is a fairly common fear, but in most cases of the men with whom I spoke, the fear dissipated as they got into the groove of the pregnancy.

There are men, albeit a relatively small number, who withdraw from their pregnant partners. Often this withdrawal is a result of a long cultural tradition that dictates that women should be kept separate from men during the nine months of gestation. Initially meant to protect and honor women, such a practice keeps men unaware of and uninvolved in the process of pregnancy. As Martin said, "During my wife's first pregnancy, I just stayed away from her. I slept in the guest room the entire pregnancy and waited outside while she delivered our son. That's what my father had done, so that's what I did." Looking back on the birth of his first child, Martin actually felt saddened by his behavior.

Below, I have culled from a number of sources some information that may be helpful in understanding just what your man is experiencing at this time. I also offer some suggestions to encourage him to become more involved:

▶ Men may feel jealous in the second trimester. Just as women experience a shift in their mental framework, so too do men. Your pregnancy is now real, and they are forced to deal with feelings of being replaced or misplaced. As one man said, "I know it was irrational, but I would experience waves of panic that my wife was never going to pay attention to me again. I just couldn't handle it." The advice of those men who have been through this experience? "Talk to him, pay attention to him, and by all means show him that you still think he is hot, hot, hot."

➤ Invite him to your OB appointment when you know an ultrasound is scheduled. This is a very intimate experience and one that makes the realness of your new baby tangible and pulls you and him together more tightly as you first witness the miracle you created together. As one woman shared, "At our first ultrasound, we got two prints of the baby—one for the refrigerator and one because my husband wanted a picture of Adam in his wallet."

➤ Involve your man in your pregnancy by letting him feel your belly. At around five or six months, the baby's movements can be felt outside the belly. Many men are shocked at how powerful it is when they first sense the baby's aliveness in this way.

➤ Some men fear that sex will hurt the baby. You need to reassure him that the baby is snugly safe in your uterus, surrounded by amniotic fluid. Many men think their penises will act like spears, able to puncture the baby. Actually, as Dr. Black sagely observed, there is no need to worry as the end (glans) of the penis is as soft as a marshmallow.

➤ Be sensitive to his sudden shyness. While all men don't experience inhibitions during pregnancy, some men do, especially about physical intimacy. You may be surprised by this news, but once you realize your man may be holding back, you might just feel the urge to initiate and seduce him more often.

➤ Encourage him to enjoy solo sex if you're not feeling sexual and you are comfortable with him masturbating. One woman said she regularly presented her husband with a couple of good erotic films. "He was so happy. I could see the relief in his eyes—I know it meant a lot to him."

Throughout your pregnancy, take the time to have talks with your man about your desire to be close to him during these months, but explain that it may not always lead to sexual intercourse. Communication here is key. Why? Because once he is past the Proud Papa stage, one of a man's biggest fears is that your sex life will never be the same or will disappear. You need to let him know the importance of him as your sexual partner. Explain that the mind may be willing but the flesh is weak. Tell him, too, that your lovemaking is going to be different right now, but not forever. You need to let him know how you feel about him, that you love him and you aren't shutting him out.

Fashion Advice for Burgeoning Moms to Be

No doubt you've noticed a few changes by now. As your body becomes more curvy—dare we call it luscious?—you need to embrace the bodaciousness and reject the associations with "fat and out of shape." It's easy to get distracted by your changing shape in a negative way—as one woman said, "Whose thighs are these, anyway?" But there are great ways to enhance your figure while pregnant.

Designers such as Liz Lange, Belly Basics, Japanese Weekend, and A Pea in the Pod are taking pregnant women out of the closet and giving women the option of wearing more formfitting, flattering, and yes, sexy clothing. And, you don't have to buy such clothes at expensive boutiques. Lori, one rather chic woman, told me that she got her entire maternity wardrobe at Target, which sells a line of Liz Lange clothing. So instead of hiding your curves, flaunt them.

I have a degree from the Fashion Institute of Technology in New York, and one piece of advice I learned and still adhere to is the importance of presentation, presentation, and presentation. Whatever your style preference or the shape of your body, make clothes work for you. You may want to keep these ideas in mind as your body changes:

- **Sexy lingerie**—It's often expensive, but it's worth it. Indulge in a few good items that make you feel good each morning when you dress. Investigate lingerie from Japanese Weekend (*www.japaneseweekend.com*), A Pea in a Pod (*www.apeainapod.com*), Victoria's Secret (*www.victoriassecret.com*), and the Gap (*www.gap.com*). The new rage in pregnancy panties are thongs made to fit just under the belly. One client swears by the low-rise thong made by Victoria's Secret. Not only will your partner thank you for it but you will enjoy your sexy silhouette.

- **Bras**—Spend the money on three really good bras that you feel good in. It is *so* worth it when you get dressed every morning.

- **Pajamas**—Get creative in bed. Your pajamas are soon going to become uncomfortable. Ribbed tanks that show off your arms and breasts offer a sexy alternative. As one woman shared, "For the first six months, I slept in XL ribbed tanks from the Gap and J. Crew, with a pair of my husband's boxers. He loved it."

- **Sweaters**—When choosing sweaters, opt for formfitting instead of bulky and shapeless. But make sure the sweater has enough length to cover your tummy region.

- **Black, black, black**—Black is not just for city girls. One woman said she went to the Gap and purchased no fewer than five pairs of black stretch pants. "They slim me down and are comfortable—and they weren't even maternity."

- **Shawls and scarves**—Make creative use of shawls and scarves. These accessories are the embodiment of femininity and can enhance your pregnancy glow with a simple soft velvet drape over your arms or shoulders—an ecru lace shawl is particularly romantic and sensual. Wear a chemise in a solid column of color, and take two color-coordinated scarves and tie their ends together on the diagonal. Let them drape asymmetrically over one shoulder and your bump when you head out in the evening. These may be the only articles of pregnancy attire you'll want to wear again after delivery.

- **Overalls**—If you do like to wear overalls for their comfort appeal, select a complementary color for skin tone and accessorize well with hair clips, scarves, bracelets, or earrings. I saw an adorable style in a Munich maternity window in which the mannequin had one shoulder clip of the overalls undone, and a sweater tied casually by the arms at an angle over one shoulder and draped across the belly.

- **Footwear**—Buy a sexy pair of shoes that make your legs look sleek and narrow but are still comfortable. But sexy shoes don't have to be high heels. There are many attractive styles with low or no heels. High heels can be a problem with your shifting balance.

- ► **Mirrors**—Choose your most flattering angles in any mirror or window. Some Hot Mamas recommend avoiding constant rear-end mirror checks—they feel there is no need to concentrate on this area.
- ► **Frumpy factor**—Avoid any outfit or style that makes you feel frumpy. As one woman said, "Shapeless muumuus can make you look like a walking duvet cover."
- ► **Posture**—Clothes hang and move better when you are most erect. I'm afraid, ladies, your mother was right, so try sitting and standing straight. At no time will good posture be more your friend than now.

No one will make you feel better about your physical presentation than you—and following a few fashion rules helps accomplish this.

Maternity Underwear Does Not Have to Be Frumpy

Even if you can't quite put yourself in a sexy thong, there are still ways to avoid the dreaded over-the-belly underpants of yesteryear. Try Land's End, Cherokee (Target's brand), and the Gap for lightly elasticized bikini briefs that are comfortable, don't give you an offensive panty line, and offer room to grow. And keep your man in mind: one woman confessed that her husband was so repelled by her over-the-belly granny underwear that he put all of hers in the freezer! Get the message?

If It's Good for Your Heart . . .

Keep exercising. It's not only good for your heart, it's good for your head. But even more important, it's also good for your sex life. The more active you remain, the more vital you will feel. You will have more energy, and your body will feel and look more toned. And chances are you will feel more sexually appealing.

In the second trimester, as your belly begins to protrude and you put on extra weight, you do need to keep in mind certain issues when you exercise: a change in your balance and your need for more fluids to stay hydrated. If you're already in shape for walking, yoga, swimming, tennis, or golf, then continue for as long as you feel comfortable. I know of several women who swear that their increased abdomens actually improved their golf games, as they lowered their center of gravity and gave them perfect spheres around which to rotate. And another woman told me that she played tennis until her third trimester. "I ran less, but hitting the ball made me feel so good."

Be aware that during sex play you should avoid abrupt movements or extreme pressure on your limbs. As your center of balance has shifted, beware of falling, stumbling, or crashing into something during a bout of passion or other athletic pursuits. Also, you may experience "the clumsies," where you drop everything. Again, this new lack of coordination can be attributed to your changing position in space.

Other tips for exercise in the second trimester:

- Continue to do your squats.
- Modify your sit-ups (or your Pilates Hundreds) by keeping your head on the floor.
- Increase your Kegels.
- Be careful during hip openers, such as pigeon in yoga, as the hormone relaxin working on your ligaments can make you feel deceptively more limber.
- Continue your light arm weights.
- Continue your pelvic tilts.
- Sit up straight and breathe more easily—your mother was right!

Celebrate Your Shape

In some circles, women are so entranced by their pregnant shapes that they decide to make molds of their pregnant bellies/bodies. One such company that offers this artistic service is *www.bellymask.com.*

Share Your Dreams

Many women and men report an increase in erotic dreams during pregnancy. As one woman said, "If my dreams are any indication, I am just brimming with desire. Last night I woke up soaking wet after having a wild dream in which my husband seduced me in our laundry room." Because their sleep patterns are changing, pregnant women tend to spend more time in REM, therefore dreaming more. Since their sleep tends to be lighter, and they wake up more easily, pregnant women often have an easier time remembering their dreams upon waking, and many of these dreams seem to have an erotic edge to them. Indeed, Angie Harmon, in a *Redbook* article, mentioned that she kept having erotic dreams about having sex with movie stars during her recent pregnancy.

And it doesn't seem to matter how long you sleep for these libidinous urges to present themselves. Hillary stated she had hugely erotic dreams even when she catnapped, dreaming of sexual encounters with her partner in unusual locales—such as the gym, the backyard, and the car. Other women told me that their dreams were just that much more vivid and memorable. As Michelle said, "I had a lot of sex with people I know—even though I'm crazy in love with my husband." Caroline told me that in her second trimester, she kept having recurring dreams of past boyfriends: "Oh, there's Freddie, and Bobby, and look—there goes Tommy. It was like a parade of every guy I had kissed and fooled around with!"

The couples who shared their dreams with their partners said they got even more mileage out of the fantasies. Some couples relish their favorite fantasies, which they visit again and again. Others expand into new territory, sometimes guided by the unexpected erotic dreams that fuel their libidos and activities. For some couples these new ideas remain staples of their play after the baby is born. With fantasies you can be more creative because pregnancy sex is inherently a sexuality of adaptation.

Here are some fantasies to try on for size:

- Have phone sex when you and your man are apart—even if you're just in different offices.
- Role-play: does he want to be the Cabana Boy to your Bored Housewife?
- Play doctor—with his equipment.
- Talk dirty—especially before little ears can hear you.
- Get a little mad: indulge each other's domination/submission fantasy.

Encouraging fantasies while you are pregnant is a great way to steam up your bedroom, especially as you physically feel more limited by what you can do. So next time you have an erotic dream, share it with your man. And encourage your man to share his with you.

Tapping into your own reservoirs of sensuality will enable you to enjoy yourself and your sexuality more intensely now and throughout your pregnancy. As you connect to your new level of energy, keep in mind that getting in the mood is essential for most women before they have sex. And the two most essential factors for getting in the mood are being relaxed and feeling good about yourself. So take the time not only to stay close to your partner but also to take care of yourself. In the next chapter, you will find more advice and tips on how to take care of yourself, specifically how to make your body—and its ever-changing form—feel stronger, healthier, and more vital. And as you know, the stronger your body is, the more sensual and sexual pleasure it is capable of creating.

5

Your Bodacious Bod

Stage Two of Your Changing Body

MOST WOMEN EXPERIENCE HUGE IMPROVEMENTS in how they feel during the second trimester. The nausea, the fatigue, the headaches, and any all-around weakness subside, often disappearing. Here is a sample of what you have to look forward to:

- Orgasms become even easier.
- Your skin clears up and actually looks incandescent (the pregnancy glow; it's real!).
- You finally start showing, which is exciting because the whole world is nice to pregnant women. (A client marveled at how many people just openly smiled at her as she walked down the street.)
- Your breasts stop aching and actually become fun again. One small-chested woman said having larger breasts was "like playing dress-up as a little girl." Remember stuffing socks in your undershirt to see how you'd look? Well, here they are, for real—show those puppies off!

And now in place of the previous three months of challenges to your sexual desire? Why, a big return of or increase in your libido, of course. Let's give a hand for Mother Nature, shall we?

But before we get to all the fun you're going to have with your partner, I do want to review what is going on with your ever-changing body during weeks thirteen through twenty-four. Some of these physiological changes may not seem to impact your sex life or sexuality directly. However, indirectly, they may be hampering your physical libido or mental attitude toward sex. To my mind, the more you understand what's going on with your body, the closer in touch with it you can be. And the more attuned you are to your body, the more likely it is you will be able to find sexual pleasure and satisfaction.

Back to my point: you need to stay sensually and sexually alive so that you can reap the sensual and sexual benefits. This attitude and willingness are at the heart of being a Hot Mama.

Loving and Accepting Your Body

I know from listening to hundreds of women that weight gain can have a huge impact on the quality of women's sexual experiences during pregnancy. But don't assume it's always negative. Christine stated, "I was huge, just huge, and my husband couldn't keep his hands off me during my second pregnancy." Many women say they find themselves able to let go of previous inhibitions about their bodies and really relax during sex for the first time ever. They no longer worry about pulling in their stomachs or hiding their thighs, as being rotund is perceived as natural and necessary, even sexy. Sandra, a model-slim woman, commented, "Finally I didn't have to worry about holding my stomach in."

Women's standards of beauty are often much harsher than men's, and many times our partners enjoy a little extra softness. And believe me, lack of inhibition is always attractive to a man. As Beth, the mother of two, said, "It didn't seem to matter what I did, I was always turned on during both my pregnancies. I could be in the shower and my hand would stroke over my nipples, and I had to get my husband and get some action fast! And boy, did he love it—he was so turned on because I was so turned on."

Sometimes pregnant women have to work harder at accepting their bodies, and hey, some of the changes are pretty dramatic and startling. Instead of continuing to doubt your appeal or attractiveness, I suggest flipping such doubts on their head by tactfully letting your man know what it is that you need during this time. Most men I know feel so badly after the first three months of seeing their women throwing up that they are just thrilled to be able to do something for them—especially if it means providing sexual services! Jane had a fabulous idea: the "no-strings-attached orgasm." As Jane recalled, "Brian would offer it very solicitously every other day or so, and in a way, it sort of became his job throughout my second trimester. He took this role really seriously—it was so cute! At a time when my whole body felt like it wasn't mine anymore and that the growing baby was demanding all my energy, I really appreciated his ability to just give something to me without expecting anything in return." When you let your man pleasure you, your doubts about your appeal will be history.

Let us not forget it is *your body* that is changing. In my opinion, it is vital to embrace your new curves and accept some of the other less appealing visible manifestations of your pregnancy. Focus on the good work your body is doing, and use this as an opportunity to explore something new: enjoying intimacy with your partner as though you are a bodacious stranger, just passing through town for a few months, willing to experience new depths of pleasure.

The Weirdest Things that Happened to My Body

Women reported many strange things happening to their bodies throughout their pregnancies. Here are some highlights:

- ➤ "My whole bikini area darkened. No amount of shaving or waxing seemed to change my skin color."
- ➤ "The hair stopped growing on my legs."
- ➤ "I lost all body odor. As my mother would say, I no longer suffered from GAPO (Gorilla Armpit Odor)."

> ▸ "After I gave birth, I couldn't bear the taste of wine, coffee, or cilantro—three tastes I have always loved."
>
> ▸ "My belly button disappeared by the time I hit the second trimester. Now it's five months later and it still seems sunken in."

Pregnancy Brain—Fact or Fiction?

By this time in your pregnancy, you may sometimes feel as if you can't remember your name or address. Don't worry: this is a real phenomenon, commonly referred to as pregnancy brain, which has very real physiological causes. Specifically, forgetfulness, shortness of attention span, and other shifts or changes in your mental awareness and acuity are common side effects of an increase in oxytocin, a hormone that increases in the second trimester and even more so late in the third trimester.

According to Dr. Jules Black, oxytocin has an amnesiac effect on the human mind. But don't fret: you are not losing your mind; it is just on hold for a bit. Dr. Black referred me to a brilliant study done in Holland in the eighties, in which scientists let loose extremely well-trained rats into a maze and then gave them a hit of oxytocin. The rats stopped in their little tracks, clueless, and couldn't figure out which direction to go. As soon as they were given the enzyme oxytocinase, which breaks down the oxytocin, the rats then took off again in mad flight to complete the maze and get their reward.

But perhaps oxytocin's most amazing effect is its ability to wipe out the memory of the adverse effects of birth. Many women at the moment of delivery are adamant—"I will never do this again!" Just a few months later, you can hear even women who have gone through the most trying of labors and deliveries having seemingly forgotten about the pain. As Kathryn explained, "I remember it being painful, but I don't remember the pain."

Despite the scientific and anecdotal evidence to the contrary, there are new studies that say pregnancy and motherhood may make women smarter and sharper. The suggestion is that "pregnancy brain" is a myth. It is only my guess that the people behind such research are trying to disprove the idea that pregnant women should be thought of as less capable or astute, which of course they aren't.

All Lubed-Up

Some ladies in their second trimester marvel at their body's production of lubricants: more saliva and increased vaginal discharge. This extra wetness between the legs is probably white or yellow, and relatively thick. It's not an infection (unless it smells foul or is irritating, in which case, call your doctor), and it can be used to your advantage. You can set aside the store-bought lubricants you use and rely on your own natural juices for a while.

If you find your increased discharge bothersome, wear a sanitary pad, avoid panty hose or nylon undergarments, and stick to cotton-crotched undies. Steer clear of irritants like scented baths, deodorant soaps, perfumes, and above all, douches.

Many women spend their pregnancies running to the bathroom frequently, as the added weight and pressure on the bladder and the increased fluid intake take their toll. As one woman said, "I didn't want to be more than twenty-five feet from a bathroom." Specifically, as the baby takes up more room in your abdomen, your bladder has decreased capacity. In addition, the progesterone has slowed down the smooth muscle function of the bladder tissue itself. It is also fairly common to have increased incidents of urinary tract infections, bladder infections, or cystitis during pregnancy. These are marked by painful urination combined with a dreadful urgency to go. To avoid triggering such reactions, try not to hold your pee, drink a lot of fluids, and be certain to urinate after intercourse. It's also important not to ignore painful symptoms, as this could cause premature labor or a low-birth-weight baby, thought this is rare. Obviously, some of this urinary urging may inhibit you to feel sexual. However, if you take steps to keep clean and maintain your hygiene, you will feel more attractive and ready for sex.

D*id You Know?*

- Anecdotally many women find that a daily cup of yogurt containing live lactobacillus acidophilus cultures (check label for contents) can dramatically reduce their incidence of vaginal yeast infection. Many ladies prefer organic yogurt, and some like the kefir probiotic drink.
- Cranberry juice creates an environment in which it is difficult for the organisms causing bladder infection to adhere to the bladder wall.
- You should continue to drink lots of fluids—especially water—to keep yourself well hydrated and to aid the flow of fluids through your system.

Can These Breasts Get Any Bigger?

The answer is yes.

One woman told me that she thought there was something wrong because her breasts stopped hurting in the second trimester. As she said, "I didn't know that this was a normal change—I was so worried that something was wrong." By the second trimester, the glandular duct system has completed developing. The fullness remains, but the pain stops. In a nonpregnant woman, each breast weighs approximately seven ounces, and by the end of pregnancy each may weigh fourteen to twenty-eight ounces! And that's not because of fat tissue; it's in preparation for milk production.

Most women love the way their breasts look—and no doubt you, too, will think your breasts look great and their shape fabulous. Now more than ever you need to give your breasts terrific support so you don't stretch the Cooper's fascia/ligaments. Once stretched, this area will have difficulty going back, so you may want to think about wearing a comfortable bra to bed to prevent sagging later on. Buy yourself a colorful, comfortable bra (cotton or underwire), and you will sleep better and look cute to boot.

This increase in size won't be the only change you and your partner notice. You may develop stretch marks on your breasts. There may be dark veins visible just beneath the skin. Your areolas may turn brown or red-brown and enlarge: each nipple contains nerve endings, muscle fibers, sebaceous glands, sweat glands, and about twenty milk ducts. A thick yellow fluid called colostrum (a vitamin-rich pre-milk) will begin to develop and sometimes leak—though this happens more in your third trimester.

When doing a breast exam or being fondled during lovemaking, you may find noticeable lumps or nodules in your breasts. Don't be alarmed: unless quite large, they are probably clogged milk ducts. If you are concerned, call your doctor.

Breast Leaks

Leakage of colostrum may be a bit disconcerting at first. Don't worry, it doesn't mean that baby is about to arrive, and your breasts are not going to start oozing milk. But do take some steps to keep your breasts and nipples healthy and happy by keeping them clean. Some women use lanolin ointment for breast-feeding to keep nipples from drying out and cracking. One woman said she always began and ended each day by washing her nipple area with a warm, wet washcloth—she thought it helped her prevent nipple blockage later, when she was nursing. If your man is into your breasts, give him the task of this gentle rubdown at night. . . . Who knows where it might lead the two of you.

Keeping Fresh

Oral hygiene is very important now because pregnant women are more susceptible to inflammation that can lead to infection (yes, it's due to that increase in blood volume!). Again, because of the increase in blood volume, all mucous membranes, including your gums, are more sensitive to bacteria and therefore infection. It's crucial that you brush, floss, and use mouthwash as usual. Brush your tongue to minimize bacteria and freshen your breath for your lover. Tongue scrapers may become your new best friend, as they remove buildup on your tongue that is responsible for bad breath and icky mouth. I know one woman who was so worried about getting gingivitis that she flossed twice a day. Keep in mind, too, that sugary foods create more bacteria in your mouth.

Let the Dentist Be Your Friend

You'll want to see a dentist at least once during pregnancy, and it's best during your second trimester. Before the hygienist begins cleaning your teeth, make sure she or he knows that you are pregnant. Decaying teeth can be a source of infection that spreads through your system, so you must not ignore problems, but even more important is regular daily care to avoid gingivitis or bleeding gums.

The Swell

In the second trimester, most likely, your body will begin to swell in areas other than your tummy. Water retention can lead to bloating of your hands, feet, and ankles. This is known as edema, and the only remedies are to rest with your feet raised or wear support hose. There is a fashion line of thigh-high support hose called Ultraline 4000, available at *www.venosanusa.com*. Surgeons recommend them for patients who have had venous or leg surgery to give great overall leg support while they are healing. They have a broad, elasticized top that fits smoothly and comfortably at the top of the leg and is cropped halfway down the foot. As one client remarked, "When I wore my black pair with a black bra, my husband told me I looked like a *Playboy* martini glass girl—except I was preggers."

With the increased blood volume in your body, there can be significant vascular changes. You may develop vascular spiders, also called telangiectasis. These are small red elevations of skin, with branches extending outward; they can occur in the face, neck, upper chest, abdomen, and arms. According to Dr. Glade B. Curtis, these spider veins develop in 65 percent of white women and 10 percent of black women and are probably caused by high levels of estrogen. Redness of palms, *palmar erythema,* may also accompany the emergence of spider veins.

Some women may begin to detect the emergence of varicose veins, which occur when the walls of blood vessels weaken. There is a pooling of old blood, and the veins fill up with the excess blood and protrude. These may be on your legs or near the birth canal or on the vulva. Sorry to say, they're likely to worsen during pregnancy, especially if you stand a lot. Again, progesterone is at work, slowing down the smooth muscle activity of the blood vessels.

Increased varicosity is a very common problem with some easy solutions:

- Wear support hose.
- Lie on your side, not your back.
- Elevate your feet whenever possible.

➤ Wear flat shoes.
➤ Don't cross your legs.
➤ Reach for that Tylenol if you still need relief.

Your veins should go down after pregnancy.

The Squirts

By your second trimester, even though the baby is only eight to ten inches long, weighing barely one pound, there is still enough extra pressure on your bladder from the growing uterus to cause what women call the squirts when they cough, sneeze, or even laugh. Some women who are still running also find themselves unable to stop a slow trickle from happening. My best advice: do Kegels. (See page 19 for details.) However, in some cases, especially for second or third pregnancies, women say that no matter how many Kegels they do, nothing seems to work. There is an outpatient surgical procedure that can address the looseness of the pelvic floor, which contributes to the squirts (see page 191).

Increased Pelvic Congestion

We know that blood and oxygen are the two main physiological components that enable our largest sexual organ, our skin—be it on our nipples, our genitals, or our lips—to feel the enhanced sensations created during sex. So when it comes to sexual and orgasmic sensation, the more of these two the merrier. And that is exactly what happens when you are pregnant. As I stated earlier, there is an increase in blood volume. During the fourth month, the increased pelvic congestion leads to a tightening at the entry of the vagina, which is often responsible for creating even better sensation for the partner. Specifically, this increased vasocongestion can impact the Pacini's corpuscles, which are the highly sensitive cells in the tissue surrounding the vaginal entry that are very responsive to pressure and vibration—we finally have a scientific explanation for why women and vibrators go together so well!

A downside of the increased pelvic congestion, which contributes to the expanded orgasmic capacity of many women, is the occurrence of varicose veins in the genitals. But worry not—these abate after pregnancy.

Quickening

A dramatic turning point during the second trimester is the very first time you feel movement inside you. This is called quickening and can usually be felt between sixteen and twenty weeks. And ladies, get this—often you will feel the baby moving inside you in reaction to something you are doing or have done: rock that baby's boat with a lovely orgasm and it may well squirm in delight. As Dr. Black says, "For the baby it feels like they are a small dinghy in a choppy sea."

Round Ligament Stretching

As noted earlier, one of the many changes the body undergoes during pregnancy is an increase in (release of) the hormone relaxin. Like it sounds, relaxin literally relaxes the ligaments of the body as a way to prepare it for labor and delivery. Many women first experience this impact of relaxin preparing the pelvic girdle for delivery when they turn over during sleep or rise too quickly, and feel a quick stabbing pain way down low, near the groin area. Other women say they do not notice any pain but do experience an increased ability to stretch. As Michelle explained to me, "Throughout my first and second trimesters, I continued to do yoga and found that, increasingly, I was able to open my chest, shoulders, and hips more widely—I had more flexibility. This felt great—I felt more expansive and limber—especially during sex."

However, sometimes such stretching can be painful. Specifically, round ligament stretching can feel like a tearing hot knife sensation lower in the front of your abdomen. Such a reaction is usually most intense in a first pregnancy. The pain associated is caused by the increasing weight of the growing baby on the uterus as the dense, thick ligaments stretch. Fortunately, the women who experience such pain say it stops around twenty weeks, when the enlarging uterus starts to rest on the bones of the pelvic girdle. You may also experience a slight pain in the ligaments one to three hours after an orgasm, associated with the retention of the blood in the pelvic girdle. Understandably, in such cases, you may find you want to limit your movements during lovemaking to avoid that sensation.

Don't Rise Too Quickly

Are you getting dizzy? This could be due to a few factors: hypotension, which is low blood pressure; exertion of pressure on blood vessels; or a rapid drop in blood pressure when you get up too quickly. Take care getting out of bed, especially after sleep or an extended period of lovemaking, or when rising from a seated position. Heat, rest, Tylenol, girdles, and exercise might also alleviate backache or dizziness.

Changes in Your Skin

As your pregnancy continues, your skin can go through some incredible transformations. Some women can avoid them, but many who are genetically predisposed will get stretch marks, also called *striae distensae*. They can appear on your breasts, hips, abdomen, or buttocks. After pregnancy they may fade, but in all likelihood they will not entirely disappear. Sadly, there is no prevention or cure. Don't let anyone tell you that steroid cream (hydrocortisone or Topicort) can help. In fact, it can do harm. Some of this cream may be absorbed into your system and could be passed on to the baby.

Another common side effect of all this growing and stretching is itchy skin. Antihistamines or cooling lotions with menthol or camphor can help, as can a wonderful shea butter massage by your loving partner.

In many women, the midline of the skin of the abdomen becomes darker, forming a vertical line called the *linea nigra*. This may look unusual, yet it is a result of the increased hormones during pregnancy, and know it isn't there to stay. Irregular brown patches called *chloasma*—also unflatteringly known as the mask of pregnancy—can appear on the face. This is nothing a little skilled application of makeup can't cover, and it is rarely permanent. Sun exposure can intensify the problem, so it's wise to use a sunscreen with SPF 15 or higher, and to wear a hat.

Unwelcome skin tags (small flaps of skin) or moles may crop up. Whenever you have a mole that changes in appearance, it is worth checking in with your doctor.

Your skin is likely to get dry and itchy. For some women it is an all-over body annoyance; others say they are itchiest in those places under the greatest amount of stretching, particularly if this is their first pregnancy. For women who are multiparous (carrying more than one fetus), itchiness is often worst when they enter their second trimester. One woman said this: "I was itchy mainly on my stomach. My husband would slather lotion on me when we went to bed, and sometimes that was all the sex we wanted."

Another skin condition some pregnant women have to contend with is acne, due to the heightened estrogen in your system. This is akin to teenage acne breakouts when you went through puberty. However, the vast majority of pregnant women say they enjoy beautiful, clear skin for most of their pregnancy.

Hemorrhoids and Other Impediments to Getting It On

Hemorrhoids, constipation, heartburn (or *pyrosis*), and unwanted body or facial hair may impede your desire to frolic in the bedroom. Some women have shared with me that during oral sex they are especially conscious of their newly acquired hemorrhoids, which are simply dilated blood vessels in or around the anus. Admittedly, they're not pretty, and they afflict 20–50 percent of pregnant women. Some measure of relief can be obtained by sleeping on your side; avoiding constipation (and not straining while doing your business); keeping up with your red-light sex therapy while driving (Kegels); taking warm sitz baths (a small basin with warm water and Epsom salts) twice daily; using witch hazel soaks or ice packs. Also, increasing your fiber intake (eat lots of fruits and veggies) will reduce hemorrhoid size and sensitivity, as well as relieve constipation. More dramatic results for constipation can come from taking prune juice and adding bran to your diet. Keep the area from vagina to rectum clean using warm soapy water after every visit to the bathroom, and be sure to practice good genital hygiene by always wiping from the front toward the back.

Choose Your Prenatal Vitamin Wisely

For those of you who experience some constipation during pregnancy, many prenatal vitamins include a stool softener.

But for those of you who don't, ask for a prenatal vitamin without a stool softener. As one woman said, "I never had an issue with constipation, but it wasn't until the pharmacist pointed out that my prenatal vitamin contained a stool softener that I knew I was taking one unnecessarily."

The Hairiness of It All

You might be enjoying long, hard nails, as well as a new thickness and luster to your hair. But there can also be the odd hair or two in undesirable places that may cause you some embarrassment: on your chin, lips, cheeks, arms, back. Also, many women find that their pubic hair is rather, shall we say, abundant. As Laura put it, "I swear I felt like the Fly. Where did these things sprout from?" Depilatories and bleach cream should be avoided, so become reacquainted with your tweezers, razor, and waxing salon to pare down unwanted hair growth. As your belly grows, certain parts of your body become blocked from your sight line. . . . This is an excellent opportunity to employ your partner's barber skills! Women have told me that waxing, always a quick-and-easy remedy for unwanted hair around the bikini line, becomes especially painful during pregnancy. As Barbara shared, "I have a high threshold for pain, but when the aesthetician stripped the tape from my upper leg, I thought I was going to jump out a window!" So be forewarned—and perhaps take a little Tylenol prophylactically. Oh, the things we can do in our quest to become Hot Mamas!

The Nose Knows

"But I can't even *breathe,* let alone have sex!" is what one frustrated woman said to me. Stuffiness, frequent nosebleeds, and allergic symptoms can increase during the second trimester as your blood volume continues to grow, congesting and swelling the porous tissue of the nose and sinus linings. Just like in your cervix, where you may be noticing increased vaginal secretions, your entire system's increased blood flow affects the mucous membranes of the nose, specifically the capillaries, causing them to soften and swell. Nosebleeds may occur more often. You might even find your allergies increase, though for some women they improve.

The stuffy nose that comes during and right after sex is not just from your positioning; it is also a direct result of the testosterone's impact on the erectile tissue in your nose. Indeed, according to Dr. Jules Black, men who frequent topless beaches are often unaware of the connection between a stuffy nose at the beach and sexual arousal. As with all things individual, the amount of nasal erectile tissue varies from person to person—some of us have more, others less.

Goodness knows, stuffiness and irritation of the nasal passages can be an impediment to sex, but there are many good, easy-to-use remedies to relieve your symptoms:

- Use a humidifier in your bedroom during the night.
- Try BreatheRight strips to open nasal passageways.
- Prop yourself up to increase air flow.
- Keep your nose tissue moist by wetting with a washcloth or a neti pot (as advertised in many yoga magazines).
- Stay away from over-the-counter drugs.
- Drink more fluids.
- Try a nasal tissue moisturizer such as Saline Nasal Gel.
- Lubricants such as petroleum jelly may also help to reduce irritation.
- Ask your physician about taking an extra 250 mg of vitamin C to strengthen the capillaries, which will also help iron absorption.

Warnings to Consider

As you stay in touch with your body and its changes, keep in mind that there are certain conditions that will prevent you from being fully sexual with your partner. There are some instances in the second trimester and beyond when sex is not OK.

PREECLAMPSIA (OR TOXEMIA)

One of the most serious conditions that preclude sex is *preeclampsia.* Preeclampsia involves the development of several symptoms at once: hypertension (elevated blood pressure), protein in the urine, swelling (*edema*), and changes in reflexes or even seizures. Be concerned only if you have two or three of these symptoms at once. On every doctor's visit, your blood pressure will be checked and your weight taken in order to monitor changes that may indicate preeclampsia. But keep in mind that this condition occurs most often during a first pregnancy or with mothers over thirty. Once again, the only cure is delivery, but getting bed rest, drinking water, and avoiding salty foods (which make you retain fluid) can help if you've been diagnosed with it. But because of the risk of seizures (*eclampsia* means "convulsion"), most physicians recommend avoiding intense sexual activity.

INCOMPETENT CERVIX

A woman who has an incompetent cervix has a painless dilation of the cervix, which occurs prematurely and usually results in the delivery of a premature baby. Such a dilation usually does not occur before the sixteenth week, but once it is diagnosed, women are told not to engage in sexual activity—especially intercourse. If detected early enough during a routine visit, cervical cerclage, a surgical procedure, is used to keep the cervix closed for the duration of the pregnancy.

Here is a listing of other symptoms you may have in the second (or third) trimester. If any of these should occur, consult your medical professional immediately:

- constant or heavy vaginal bleeding
- blinding headaches
- severe abdominal pain
- gushing of fluid from vagina (trickle or continual wetness)

➤ high fever (more than 101.6°F) or chills
➤ severe vomiting
➤ blurring of vision
➤ painful urination

If you encounter any or all of the above symptoms, consult your health care provider. He or she may want you to abstain from sex.

Many women feel as if their bodies become machines during pregnancy. And to some extent they are: they need constant attention, fuel, maintenance, and a good lube job to run properly and smoothly. But unlike machines, women's bodies are soft, pliable, and very much an extension of their minds and hearts. In the next chapter, you will learn how other Hot Mamas connected emotionally and physically with their men during the sexual oasis of the second trimester.

6

Playing in Your Sexual Oasis

A RE YOU READY? You have more energy, your nausea is gone, and you are ready to take that renewed sensuality and rev those sexual engines—yours and your man's. Marcy said, "I suddenly felt like a kid in a sexual candy store. Once the exhaustion, nausea, and concern of miscarriage subsided, I couldn't wait to have fun again." Dana explained it this way to me: "I was so worried during the first three months that I didn't want to do anything sexual. I was like, 'Stay away from me.' Then when I got into my fourth month, my partner and I were like damn rabbits. There was no stopping us." Yet another woman, Georgia, said she and her husband were so relieved because they no longer had to deal with birth control, they just couldn't get enough of each other. "We were both so confident—I was proud of my belly, and he was so proud of being the man—we just got so into each other sexually!"

The sexual excitement of the second trimester is real, palpable, and yours for the taking and the making. Let's get to it! The tips and positions that follow are meant to take advantage of that bodacious bod and the energy resurgence of the second trimester. However, if you don't feel remarkably different—or better—and still want to take things slowly, then you can be just as happy snuggling. Or you can look ahead at some of the comfort sex tips for the third trimester described in Chapter Nine.

Look for That Libido

There is a separation between mental and physical desire, especially during pregnancy. Therefore, it can take longer for women to connect to or pay attention to their libidos. Don't wait to find yourself in a sexual swirl. By taking the initiative and getting in touch with your libido by looking for it, you will not have to wait in vain for that pilot light to turn on. Here are some ways that you can take the sensual and turn it into something sexual:

- Explore your new body with your man. While you are introducing him to your new hills and valleys, he will likely be introducing you to new sensations. Let and perhaps ask him to watch, touch, taste, and lick your swelling areolae and nipples.
- Experiment with a vibrator. Since many women say it takes longer to climax during pregnancy, a vibrator can do wonders for tired fingers and tongues. You may also want to bring out those toys you haven't played with in a while.
- Get slithery with a sensual massage.
- Watch an erotic movie—either on cable or by renting one from a video store. If you are too shy to rent one in public, go online and rent, or consult Violet Blue's wonderful compendium, *The Ultimate Guide to Adult Videos* (San Francisco: Cleis Press, 2003) which has an extensive list of Web addresses in its resource section. One film, from a private archive, entitled *Fullness*, beautifully depicts a full range of sensual sex between a married pregnant couple. There are also Web sites specializing in many forms of erotic pregnancy sex, be it oral, penetrative, or phone sex. One such site is *www.bunsintheoven.com*.

Men Have Their Own Issues

Ladies, it's important to keep in mind some of the pressures and stress your man may be under during your pregnancy, especially in the third trimester. According to Dr. Marc Ganem's study, some men can suffer from premature ejaculation and troubles with erection. Such issues tend to crop up when men first feel the fetus move within the woman's womb or have the feeling or fear of being overlooked or replaced in their partner's affections (by the soon-to-be-born baby). Other causes include a decrease in frequency of sex or abstinence, age (over forty years old), or a physiological condition (such as diabetes or hypertension) that hinders sexual functioning. However, Dr. Ganem reassures that in most cases, such negative changes in functioning are transitory in nature.

Manual Manna

Before they return to direct penetrative intercourse, many couples expand their manual sex repertoire. Indeed, it often encourages them to test new sexual waters. Besides, why not take advantage of all that wonderful lubrication you've been building? You may want to remind your man to be sure to wash his fingers, as the natural salt in their sweat can make a woman's genitals feel like they are burning, and you don't want to risk introducing any unfriendly bacteria into you.

Figure 11 shows a seminar favorite for pre-, during, and post-pregnancy. The beauty of this position is that either partner can be in the front and still feel the full length of the heat of the other partner's chest and abdomen behind.

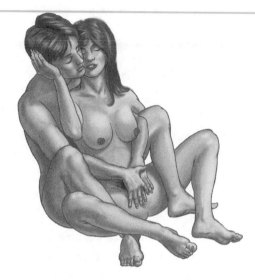

Fig. 11

Rather like spooning while sitting up, this position can be used easily outside the bedroom. This is also good if the lady still has tender breasts. Should the lady prefer to be behind so she can stimulate him, she can use a pillow to pad the breast area, to level the pressure and/or protect her breasts if they are too tender. In either case both partners can attend to the partner in the front, whether they want to do themselves, do things à deux, or just be held and relax into the partner's ministrations.

Two Manual Moves for Him

Lest we forget our male friends, I have included two manual moves with which you can pleasure your man—Basket Weave and Heartbeat of America. These are both seminar favorites, so my guess is that you will find him absolutely delighted to partake!

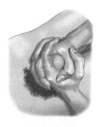
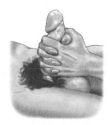
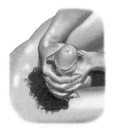

Fig. 12a   *Fig. 12b*   *Fig. 12c*

BASKET WEAVE

The ease and intensity of this two-handed technique has made it a seminar favorite.

> ***Step 1****: Clasp your warm and well-lubricated hands together as seen in figure 12a, and lower them over his erect penis with a gentle, firm downward stroke. The pressure you hold him with is such that you want the skin of his penis to "know" each ridge of your fingers and palms.*
>
> ***Step 2****: Your hands are creating on his penis the sensation of an impostor vagina that will mimic the heat, the moisture, and the pressure-filled world that is the vagina for a man's penis.*
>
> ***Step 3****: As depicted in 12b and c, once you have lowered your warm, lubricated, clasped hands to the bottom of his shaft, start a continuous up-and-down twisting motion, much like a large figure eight, as you move with a vertical stroke going from base to head.*

THE HEARTBEAT OF AMERICA

> ***Step 4****: Heartbeat of America is an up-and-down, two-handed, slow, no-twisting vertical pulsing stroke whereby your hands mimic your pulsing and contracting PC muscle tightening around his shaft. It's best done in position 12a with no twisting.*

Positions for a Slow Reentry

Couples who have had the triple whammy of fatigue, tenderness, and nausea often ease back into sex gently and start with the more gentle reclining positions.

Figures 13 and 14 illustrate two options couples give as their favorites. In both, the woman is able to experience the sensations more subtly and more gently, as they may be more intense than she has felt previously.

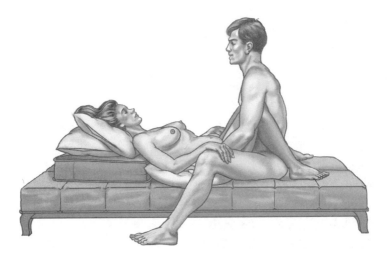

Fig. 13

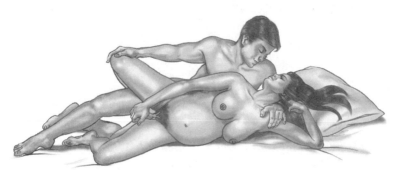

Fig. 14

In figure 13 the man is able to enjoy watching her expression and to see her breasts move with his actions. Because his feet are on the ground, he is able to use the greater stability and strength of his thighs to make his moves more finessed while maintaining complete insertion. As Kathy said, "My husband and I discovered this move by adding the ottoman to the end of his chair. All of a sudden we had a 'sex toy' bed in the middle of our great room."

Are You in Sexual Trouble or Are Things Just Different?

Many men say they feel their orgasms are premature during their partners' pregnancies. However, keep in mind that often a man's ejaculation is measured relative to the time it takes for the woman to achieve optimum stimulation. And since her arousal and full stimulation often take longer during pregnancy, it might be perceived that he climaxes too soon, when in fact, she needs more time, and he's doing what he normally does.

Introducing Toys

And speaking of sex toys, position 14 is also ideal for those couples who enjoy the more portable style of sex toys. In this position, the woman's leg over his thigh allows him easier access during penetration and to be able to create greatest sensation for her. The more open she is, the more the skin is stretched, which will contribute to her feeling the stimulation even more.

Position 14 also allows for more ease when stimulating her as intensely as she prefers, either manually or with assistance. By using his lower arm to support himself while holding her shoulder, he can cradle her neck and head. It's a great place to be for follow-up kissing.

My online survey of pregnant couples showed it is very unlikely couples will introduce toys or new items during a pregnancy. However, if toys are already an established part of their sexual routine, pregnant couples will incorporate more of them as certain positions become more difficult to manage. She can angle a vibrator or a toy to exactly where she prefers, and he can remain tightly inside of her, feeling her orgasmic contractions.

Oral Sex

Oral sex has become a standard in most couples' sexual repertoire. As Isabelle told me, "My orgasms were so great during my pregnancies—especially those from oral sex. And as it turned out, it was the first time we could do a 69 and have it work for both of us. Woo hoo!" Lori reported with pleasure that although she took longer to reach climax, her orgasms from oral sex were much deeper. As she explained, "Generally speaking I can come lickety-split—no pun intended. I found that it took me longer, but when I did, it was simply profound. I also ejaculated right before coming—all the time! My husband was like, "What is this? Nectar from the pregnancy gods?"

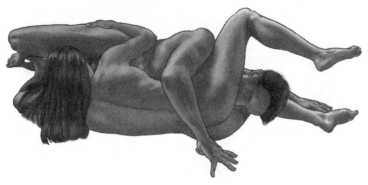

Fig. 15

Position 15 shows a couple mutually stimulating each other while on their sides. If the woman is on her side, she can support her roundness with the floor. You can do this move with pillows for support. In this side position, he doesn't have as much of her anus right on his nose. And as shown in Figure 15, he can also use her thigh as a soft pillow so he doesn't get a sore neck.

Rounding the Belly and Other Nuances

These positions are for those couples who prefer a more upright style of intercourse due to indigestion or when pressure on her breasts or abdomen is too much. Positions 16, 17, 18, and 19 give you a range of ideas for women who prefer female superior positions that allow for control of the motion and stimulation.

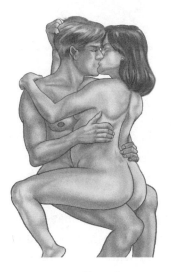

Fig. 16

Position 16 is a nonpenetrative, seated option, in which the woman can use her legs for strong up-and-down leverage along her partner's thighs for more intense clitoral stimulation. At the same time, she maintains strong firm frontal contact and kissing with her man.

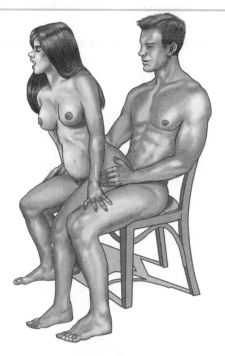

Fig. 17

Position 17 incorporates the strength of her legs and both of their arms to guide her while she is facing away from him. This gives the woman the ability to concentrate on her own sensations and go into her own world. He will be using a firm connecting hold on her hips. This is a favorite for those couples who know they can heighten their orgasmic experience when large muscle masses, such as their thighs, are contracting at the same time as the orgasmic buildup.

Figure 18 shows a couple who choose a more elevated reclining position supported by pillows and cushions. The woman is using the strength of her arms to maintain or increase the angle she prefers. The Liberator® Ramp can also be used for this position.

Position 19 illustrates a similar lower-body-elevated position supported by the Liberator® Wedge, with a greater back-angled seated position for a woman who chooses a more front-vaginal-wall form of

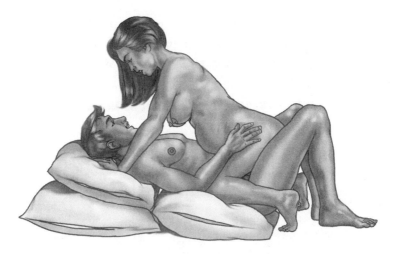

Fig. 18

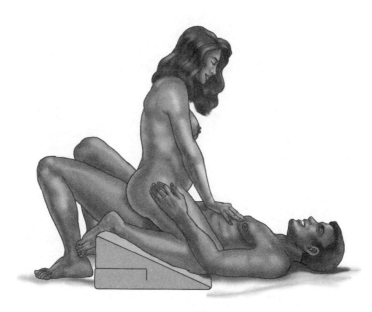

Fig. 19

stimulation. Using the Liberator® Wedge, both partners can concentrate on sensation rather than maintaining their places.

The use of legs makes positions 20 and 21 favorites during mid- and later pregnancy, as there is reduced pressure on the lady's stomach and it's easy for the woman to adjust her position.

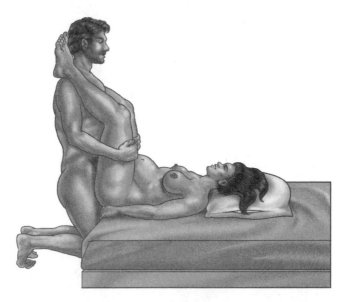

Fig. 20

In 20 she is holding the edge of the chaise while using the strength of her legs with her heels over his shoulder to position herself as she chooses. "Lying on my back while he entered me became a 2112 (our address) special when we were having our first. It was like I could feel him filling me up." In this lower kneeling position, his thighs up against the firm backs of her thighs allow him to easily maintain position without too much shifting.

In 21 the lady prefers more of a front connection with her man and wraps her legs around him. Yet due to her angle supported by pil-

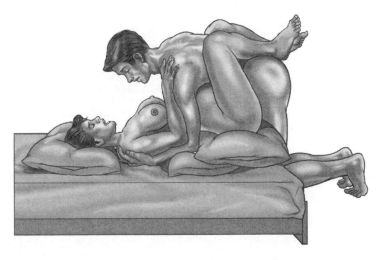

Fig. 21

lows, which raise her hips, she doesn't have to be concerned about pressure on her tummy while still being as close to him as possible.

G Spot

Due to the increased vasocongestion during pregnancy, some women find their G spot increases in size and sensitivity. Figures 22, 23, and 24 illustrate different styles of G spot and AFE (anterior fornix erotic) zone stimulation. Kathryn said, "I think [my G spot] got bigger—from the supposed size of a dime to that of a silver dollar. I absolutely loved it when my husband stimulated my G spot with his finger while he went down on me—yowee, that was a release."

In 22 the man on his knees has his thighs braced by the end of the bed. With her hips raised by a pillow to meet his groin, the man need only use short thrusts to hit the perfect spot of the woman who knows the best angle for her G spot.

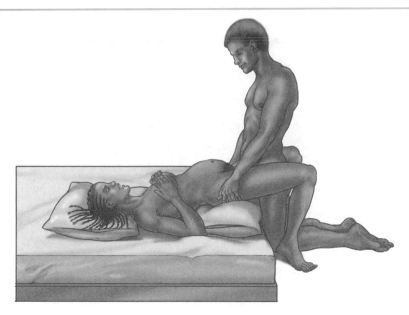

Fig. 22

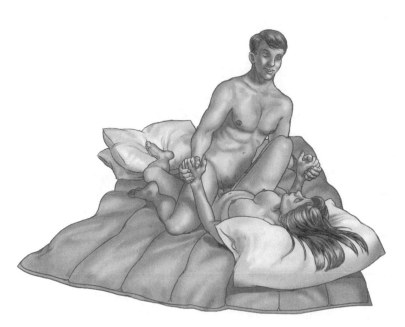

Fig. 23

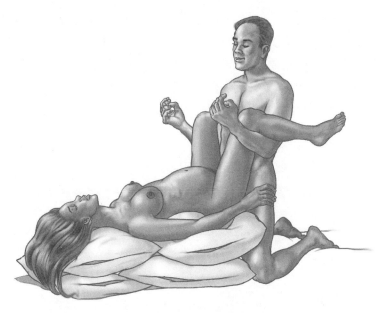

Fig. 24

Figure 23 shows the option for those who know her most sensitive internal zone is more on one side. They can use the combined strength of their arms to position the motion of the firm upward stroke they prefer.

Figure 24 shows a man using the strength of his upper arms to lift the woman to her preferred angle, while he uses short pelvic thrusts along the front vaginal wall to strongly stimulate her G spot. She can adjust the angle by flexing her thighs to lift her pelvis, which will also result in tightening the vaginal entry for him. This position also creates very strong glans (head of penis) stimulation for him.

Rear Entry

Rear entry can remain a staple of many couples' sexual diet throughout the pregnancy. As Miranda said, "I just found it more comfortable for my husband to enter me from behind. I would place a soft pillow under my stomach and widen my knees and legs. It felt so good to be penetrated that deeply."

Most women do need to make such adjustments for their growing tummy and its weight at the end of the second and into the third trimester.

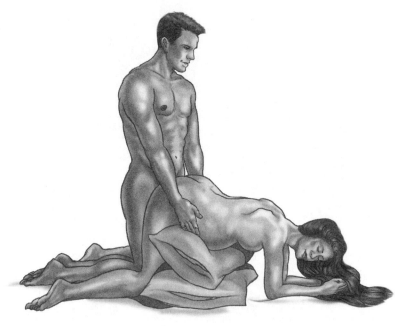

Fig. 25

Figure 25 shows a variation on a theme, in which the lady is comfortably supported by pillows, but it could just as easily be over the end of an ottoman, the bed, or the Liberator® Shape ramp. Invariably, the determining factor for this position is the size of her stomach, as well as finding a forward bend position that is comfortable for her.

Standing Positions

For those couples who enjoy standing positions, please be aware that the major body changes throughout your pregnancy will impact your balance and center of gravity; hence you will need to adjust and adapt.

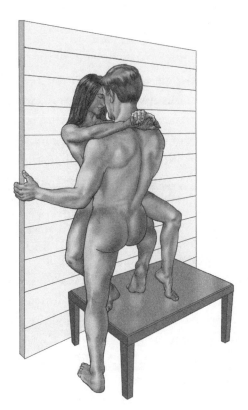

Fig. 26

Holding on to a solid stationary surface is necessary to maintain balance. If you enjoy standing positions, you may want to take advantage of them now because your increasing size is likely to interfere with any kind of the standing favorites until after you deliver, when your center of gravity isn't so impacted. Here we see a couple using a strong table as partial support for the lady while she is firmly held by her man, who maintains balance and position by holding the side of the wall. For those who say, "Standing positions—no way!" I will share one couple's comment: "It might not take that long—it has that 'quickie' feeling."

Anal Sex

Many women who experience pain or too much sensitivity in their vaginas discover anal sex as a wonderful option when they, or their partners, want penetration. And for women who have *placenta previa* (see page 46), the anus can become a new erogenous zone. As Dr. Jules Black points out, "Anal intercourse and stimulation are experienced much more frequently by women than is generally acknowledged. The rectum is being called upon to play more than an alimentary role and is also widely used for sexual purposes." He also shared that a client with placenta previa, who was prohibited from having vaginal penetration, found anal sex "eroticized" that area of her body—which until then she'd not discovered. And the owners of New York City's famed Toys in Babeland write in their book, *Sex Toys 101,* "Intense sexual gratification is the number one reason people have anal sex. Anal sex can send the turn-on meter through the roof."

As I've mentioned and addressed in all my previous books, there are still people for whom anal sex is taboo, based on two myths: that a woman who has anal sex is only doing it to please her boyfriend and that men who enjoy anal sex are closet homosexuals. Nothing could be further from the truth. Again the gals from Toys in Babeland quite nicely spell out the reasons to try "butt sex":

1. A whole lot of people swear it feels great.

2. It is part of your genitals, and you owe it to yourself to explore it.

3. There is no pain involved.

4. Variety is the spice of sex.

5. Guys: It's the only route to your very own G spot.

6. Women: It's another route to yours.

7. Closed-minded bigots think it's a sin, so it must be fun.

8. Your anus is a part of yourself you can choose to enjoy.

9. Sex is a playground for adults.

10. Why not?

There are four major positions for anal sex:

1. Missionary, with woman on bottom

2. Woman on top

3. Doggie style

4. Spooning*

As always, if you are not comfortable with anal play, then don't do it. If you are prevented from having penetrative intercourse for the duration of your pregnancy (on doctor's orders), then there are numerous other ways to feel pleasure and give pleasure. Begin by staying connected to your partner, so that there is no room for distance to grow. Keep talking—about what you want and what you can't wait to do once the baby is born. And remember, enjoy yourselves.

The second trimester offers tremendous room for many options for sexual pleasure. Most women find themselves being creative in terms of discovering new positions as they adjust themselves for sex with a belly, and most men love this added spice. As you enter your third trimester, you may begin to feel a bit more hampered by that growing belly—but have no fear, you can still find multiple ways to continue enjoying great connecting sensuality and, should you choose, that wildly delicious orgasm!

*Venning, Rachel and Cavanah, Claire, *Sex Toys 101*, Simon & Schuster, New York, 2003.

The Third Trimester

7

The Final Frontier

MOST PREGNANT WOMEN I have encountered find that after the exciting physical and emotional roller-coaster ride of their first two trimesters, these last three months offer something entirely different. As their bodies grow more massive (even the slightest woman will be amazed at her capacity to expand), the pace of life slows down somewhat. Rushing through your day seems anathema to you now as you need to lumber your way upstairs and downstairs, from one activity to the next. You just can't move fast.

This newly languid way of operating can be liberating in the bedroom, enabling you to truly enjoy prolonged erotic moments and savor the small things. It's not about excitement and penetration anymore; it's about a more profound sensual, even spiritual, enjoyment and relaxation. As twenty-seven-year-old Stephanie said to me, "After six months of no wine, no intense biking (I was a die-hard biker), and no sushi, sex was the only fun thing I still had, and boy did I take advantage of it!"

In essence, this chapter is devoted to helping you and your partner chart the very intense period leading up to the birth of your child. You naturally slow down, especially by your thirty-fifth or thirty-sixth week. The reality of parenthood is also settling in. You have probably spent a considerable amount of time nesting, preparing your new baby's room, especially if you are first-time parents. If throughout the first two trimesters, you have been staying closely connected, sharing plans and wishes for the future, revisiting your past as you head toward this new phase in your life, then you will find this final frontier an opportunity for even more intimacy. And though some of you may not feel so randy, staying physically close to your partner at this time can be enormously comforting. Indeed, sex in the third trimester is most often about comfort and connection.

Checking in with Your Priorities

The third trimester is often about planning for the immediate and not so immediate future. With that in mind, I want to bring your attention to how quickly establishing priorities can be confused with applying pressure. Each woman is unique, and each couple is unique in the relationship, whether we are talking about how the partners met, how they argue, or how they make love. And what is right for one person is not necessarily right for someone else. If another person's experiences/looks/behaviors resonate for you, then that should be your test as to whether the same may work for you. However, if some advice doesn't ring true for you, then you have every right to disregard it.

The world of pregnancy is one of so many physical, mental, and emotional changes that the last thing a pregnant woman needs is *more* pressure. There is this ridiculous pressure to do everything right: gain the right amount of weight; choose the right delivery style; buy the right baby clothes; select the right nursery, the best maternity leave, the right baby nurse, etc., etc. This pressure is often unspoken, although with some relatives and friends it may be more obvious, but the point is they are not in your relationship with your partner or your baby—*you* are, and you have full permission to set your priorities as you choose.

So as you begin to mentally and physically prepare for the arrival of your little one (or ones, as the case may be), do yourself a favor and keep in touch with what works best for you—especially when it comes to having sex and staying intimate with your partner.

I asked Dr. Jules Black, one of my expert consultant ob-gyns, when he thinks a woman should stop having sex, and his response was fairly straightforward: "When your contractions are ten minutes apart, push him off and tell him to get you to the hospital!" Seriously, though, what his response actually tells you is that when you have a clean bill of health and no complications, your sex life need not be interrupted until delivery.

Similar to how you may have felt in your first trimester, being sexual in the third trimester is more about a mental willingness and openness to sex and intimacy than an overt need or desire to be sexual. As one woman explained, "Toward the end I felt like a whale, sitting on a couch with a rash on my inner thighs. And even though sex may have been on my mind, it was awkward to bring it up. All I wanted to do was pay attention to our relationship. I wanted to connect, I wanted to feel something was familiar, because God knows there was very little left in my life that felt that way, and also we had so little time left when it would be just the two of us. I wanted to take full advantage of that." Another woman explained how she and her husband relied on their sense of humor. "Thank God we had a great sense of humor because at this point I would have to be on top, and the baby moving around was like a scene out of *Alien*. There would be times we would be laughing so hard at the baby, we'd have to start all over again, which wasn't such a bad thing."

For other couples, the closer to the delivery date they got, the more sex became "too much like a gymnastics event," and they chose to maintain their intimacy via nonpenetrative sex or simple cuddling. The upside of expanding your sensual and sexual options is you will then have more to draw from after the baby is born.

But as I've been saying throughout these pages, when you decide to stop having sex is up to you.

Are You Familiar with Camiknickers?

If your thighs are sensitive from chafing, try using cami-knickers. These are not only sexy but useful. What are they? They are like long silk shorts that stop the inner thighs from rubbing together—imagine flappers at the beach. There is a new line of hose called Mama Spanx, which are available at *www.spanx .com*, Saks Fifth Avenue, Nordstrom, and high-end boutiques.

Increasing Your Intimacy

For a lot of couples, these nine months can be life changing for more reasons than just creating a baby—including the intimacy that comes from planning your future together. This is also another time to keep your man in the loop. Keep him abreast (no pun intended) of all developments—physical, emotional, and mental. And ladies, now is another time to consider your man's experience of your pregnancy. According to Dr. Marc Ganem, there are a number of changes in the man's sexuality during pregnancy based on the following parameters:

- His desire may shift throughout the nine and a half months, depending on how sex was before the pregnancy, the number of pregnancies his partner has had, his age, and how informed he is about the realities of sex during the pregnancy.
- Men are usually very motivated to make adjustments during your pregnancy in order to stay sexually connected.
- Men enjoy sexual touch. Massage and erotic touch have a twofold mission: to maintain and reassure the couple of their sexual dialogue, even if it is only touching, and to maintain the erotic awareness of the body.

The more sexually connected you stay as a couple throughout your pregnancy, the healthier your relationship will be—now and in the future. I refer to Dr. Phil McGraw's statement at the beginning of his book *Relationship Rescue,* in which he comments that a couple's sexual intimacy is "one of a very short list of things that distinguishes their particular relationship from others. . . . There must be a sexual bond between the two of you, a kind of chemistry that makes you two recognize that you are more than friends who share a life. You are mates." With that in mind, a simple word of caution: those couples who have no or little sexual or sensual contact during pregnancy risk separation. As Dr. Marc Ganem found in his study, "The period after the birth of a child is a crucial one in which couples have to learn a new eroticism between the two partners. But it is also a time of many dangers, the numbers of which are so impactful. Many couples separate in a year or two after the birth of the child."

It's therefore very important to continue to increase your intimacy with your partner. Think about this as creating a cocoon-like feeling between the two of you. Only the two of you can really experience the specialness of this time. One couple shared with me that though the woman was too uncomfortable physically to have sex, they did a lot more cuddling. "Vincent was just so much more affectionate. He would wrap himself around me as we lay side by side on our bed or on the couch. He was much more attentive—he would bring me things to eat and drink. Simple things, but they made me feel so much better, so much closer to him."

Nesting

Have you found yourself cleaning closets? Becoming fixated on your linen closet? Most women go through such a phase when they are preparing their nest for the arrival of a new baby. Obviously some of this planning and preparing is just common sense. But what I have gleaned from speaking to women directly about their nesting instinct is how real and subliminal it feels to them. Indeed, Dr. Jules Black says that nesting is one of a distinct number of phenomena that precede the onset of labor. For those women having their first child, the graph below* shows the specific physiological and emotional events that occur, in a variety of sequences, one to three days before labor begins:

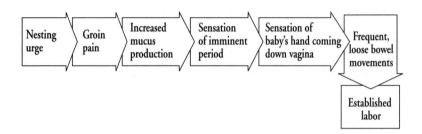

Dr. Black then points out that in subsequent pregnancies, these phenomena happen at an even faster pace or even simultaneously, spaced over one or two days. He says, "I have even known women who have experienced each and every phenomenon over a time as short as two or three hours!"

My point in bringing up the urge to nest in the context of your sexuality is that as you finish your third trimester, your body and your mind are focused on one thing: delivering your baby. If, by chance, you notice a dip in your interest in being sexual, there is a good reason for it!

Cultivating Humor When You're Feeling Rather Humorless

OK, so you can barely sleep at night, and you may be snoring so badly that your husband or partner has left you alone in your queen-size bed, preferring the sofa in the living room. And getting on your feet in the morning takes about ten minutes. Never mind the frustration of no longer being able to see beyond your swollen hands to your feet—have no fear! You are still a wonderful, sexy woman.

Let me ask you a quick question: are you laughing or crying at this point? I hope you're laughing. At this stage of pregnancy, there is no

*Black, Jules, *Body Talk*, Angus & Robertson Publishers, North Ryde, Australia, 1988.

avoiding the physical limitations. As many of the respondents in my online survey declared, their sense of humor was a huge factor in being able to navigate the tension and nerves that start to build in the third trimester as you get closer and closer to labor and delivery.

A playful attitude is the best medicine when you begin to feel weighed down. As one woman said, "I was pregnant from my earlobes down to my toes. I couldn't move, but I could nest on the couch with my hubby, and that was as much moving as I wanted to do. Long card games became our nightly ritual." Another couple went dancing. As Frances said, "We love to dance after a Friday or Saturday dinner. Now instead of dancing face-to-face with my husband, we dance with him behind me, his arms wrapped around and holding me and the baby."

When things start getting a bit tense, here are some suggestions for lightening the mood:

- Go to the movies. Heaven knows, this will be difficult once Junior arrives. You may want to stay away from violent or gory films and choose instead lighthearted, romantic, or intellectually stimulating movies.
- Go out to dinner. Have someone cook for you. Don't clean up. Enjoy the ritual of dining out with your lover before he becomes a papa and you a mama.
- Invite friends over. If you don't want to cook, then order in or ask your friends to bring potluck.
- Play Twister or go out dancing. OK, I'm only half-serious, but do you get my point? Have fun and don't take your physical limitations too seriously. Move to your new groove even if you can't exactly manage a salsa, a tango, or a bunny hop.

Little Preparations That You Will Relish

Although your third trimester is an extended meditation on getting to the finish line, it really is just the starting point of a whole new whirlwind. In the days and weeks immediately following the arrival of your little one, you'll have more visitors than you'll probably care to, and one thing that will help you feel better is if you actually feel presentable during those visits.

Most women say they can just tell when they are nearing labor. If you sense delivery is soon, and you still feel up to it, you might want to do some or all of the following because heaven knows you won't have the time or energy to do them for quite a few weeks after. As soon as one of my clients arrived at the hospital, she had her husband call her beauty salon. Her request? To send over someone immediately to the labor/delivery room so she could be waxed before giving birth!

Her are some other suggestions:

- Get your hair cut (nothing radical; just go for a basic maintenance trim).
- Get a bikini wax (yes, it will hurt, but doesn't it always?).
- Shave or wax your legs and underarms.
- Tweeze your eyebrows.
- Get a manicure and pedicure—as the baby's arrival approaches, you may want to simply buff your nails and forgo the polish.
- Get a massage (prenatal, of course)—pampering will be on the back burner for you for a while very soon.

You may also want to do a little extra shopping—not for the baby, but yourself. What you are looking for—either at some of the stores mentioned herein or online—is comfortable, attractive loungewear that you can live in. Remember that most women don't even leave the house for at least two weeks after having a baby, so loungewear is perfectly fine when you greet all your friends and family who arrive with baby gifts. One of my girlfriends neglected to do this and as a result lived in her husband's ratty flannel shirt and her baggy maternity leggings. Looking back at all the pictures from that first week—there are always lots of pictures that first week—she now cringes at how she looks for posterity!

But now is not the time to go shoe shopping, because your feet have likely expanded. However, you will definitely want to be comfortable with that extra weight on them. Here are some suggestions for footwear from the field:

- ballet shoes with support inserts
- thick-soled flip-flops
- fur-lined boots such as Uggs
- Dansko clogs
- comfy slippers around the house or apartment

Find a nice robe, some cute sweats, new pajamas—whatever you think you will feel comfortable and presentable in. (If you plan to breast-feed, remember to get shirts that button down the front and some nursing bras). One savvy mother presents all her mom-to-be friends with a long dark-colored velour robe that zippers down the front and washes easily. Her comment: "You're sore, you're oozing, and you will live in this thing! Zip it off after three weeks!" I truly believe that we heal faster when we psychologically feel better, so looking good during this time has its medical advantages, as well.

Waxing Tips from One Who Should Know

This is advice from Nance Mitchell, a Los Angeles–based aesthetician for the stars: "I usually tell women if they have never been waxed before to not do it just before they deliver. There is a lot more hair, and that area has a lot more blood in it, and the area is more sensitive. If they have been 'groomed' throughout their pregnancy, I do smaller strips. Some clients who know they are having a C-section will request that I take off all their hair. This is true for other women, as well, so they don't have to shave. I have had clients who were in labor stop by on their way to the hospital to be done. They want to make sure they don't have to worry about this afterward."

There is no doubt that your third trimester is filled with anticipation. As you feel your baby move inside of you, the reality that he or she is soon arriving is hard to ignore. As movement becomes more cumbersome, and your body prepares more immediately for childbirth, sex may seem to be the last thing on your mind. In the next chapter, you will see more about what's happening inside your body. As you consider these final-inning changes, do consider that sexual and sensual comfort do not have to go completely by the wayside.

The Body Resplendent
Stage Three of Your Changing Body

YOUR BODY HAS SLOWED DOWN; your belly continues to grow. This is all part of where your body is during your third trimester. As we take a close look at what's happening inside of your body, keep in mind that although you can think of nothing but delivering your tiny bundle of joy, there are ways to enjoy these final three and a half months of pregnancy through sexual and sensual comfort. But before we jump into bed, so to speak, let's take a look at what is happening in that magnificent body of yours.

Your Body During the Third Trimester

By the third trimester, you are going to slow down. Your baby is gaining considerable weight with each passing week, which is the main reason for this slowing pace. Getting in and out of bed takes longer, walking to and from your car takes longer, even eating can take longer. Women generally gain about a pound each week, and even when you swear you cannot possibly expand any more, you will continue to get bigger. And though moving around is now more cumbersome than ever, sex is still possible—though with considerably more supportive enhancements (as you will see in the next chapter).

Indeed, many women told me that in the two weeks moving from second to third trimester, they felt a similar kind of exhaustion to what they experienced in their first trimester. Allyson related, "I could not make it through the day without taking a nap. I was exhausted, and it kind of scared me—then a friend of mine who is about two weeks ahead of me said that she had gone through the same thing, and that it passed. Well, it did—thank God." Although some women never felt this change in the degree of their tiredness, all the women with whom I spoke said that after thirty weeks, they needed more rest.

In the first three-quarters of the third trimester, your baby will become more active. Many women say they can feel their babies turning over, kicking, punching, and moving from side to side. As you approach your due date, however, and the baby almost fills your entire abdomen cavity, this activity tends to slow or cease, as there is increasingly less room for the baby to move.

Some women also experience false labor, or Braxton Hicks contractions, which have nothing to do with labor. Although such light, nonpainful contractions with no rhythm can occur throughout pregnancy, they tend to increase in your third trimester. But again, some women don't experience them at all.

Mysterious Leaks of the Final Inning

As you have probably noticed by now, it is common, though perhaps annoying, to have increased discharge and urine leakage during this stage of pregnancy. You may find that coughing, laughing, sneezing, or relaxing during lovemaking causes some incontinence. This is where your Red Light Sex Therapy—Kegels!—will prove indispensable. This type of stress incontinence is noticeably different from a rupture of the amniotic sac. Sheila was three weeks away from her due date when she told me this story: "We had just moved into our new house, and it was very hot. At about one P.M., I began to feel small contractions and a gush of liquid. I immediately assumed I was in labor, so we rushed over to the hospital. After the nurse checked to see if I was dilating (I wasn't), she hooked me up to an IV for fluid. I asked her, 'Didn't my water just break?' And the nurse very kindly said, 'No, honey, you just peed in your pants.' It turns out that I had become dehydrated, which brought on Braxton Hicks contractions."

Be aware that dehydration can bring on actual contractions and premature labor.

Women assure me that you will know when your water breaks. "I could have filled a bathtub; as it was, I soaked our entire queen-size bed," remembers Tracy. If you feel a gush of liquid and see a leaking of clear, yellow, green, or bloody fluid, do not have intercourse. Call your doctor, as your water may have broken. As one woman recalled, "I was brushing my teeth, and I felt fluid run down my leg. Goodness knows, there had been so many different body sensations and changes that had happened during my pregnancy that I assumed I was just peeing. So I called my mother-of-three girlfriend, who said, 'Girl, you are in labor.'"

A *Reminder on Piercings*

Ask your doctor about removing labial piercings during delivery and reinserting directly afterward. Try threaded or circular barbells in your nipples, as these can easily be removed for breastfeeding. Never breastfeed with body jewelry in place! It is a choking hazard and could cause infection. Dr. Jules Black actually recommends removing your piercings during the start of the second trimester before things get too stretched out.

Hot and Heavy

Regardless of the temperature outside, most women sweat so much during these last days, you may think of yourself as living in your own personal sauna. This heat factor definitely comes into play during sex, so you may want to watch that you do not overheat during more passionate moments. But a hot and heavy session with your lover cannot raise your body temperature for long enough to be of danger to your fetus.

A pregnant woman's metabolic rate—the rate at which her body expends energy at rest—rises by 25 percent, so increased sweating is to be expected. The point here is you might want to refrain from going on a long hike in extreme heat, so you don't lose fluids rapidly and create a cause for concern. It's always important to stay well hydrated. Remember the woman mentioned previously who brought on contractions from dehydration!

Word *to the Wise About Taking Baths*

- Be careful getting in and out of the bathtub—use those railings.
- Don't make the water too hot. Most doctors warn against elevating your body temperature. A good rule of thumb: if you are comfortable, your baby is comfortable. Don't let yourself start sweating in the bathtub!
- Do not take a bath if your water has broken. Sponge bathe instead to clean yourself.

Sex and Infections

There is little documented link between sexual activity and an increase in infections during pregnancy. However, this changes by the final month, when the protective amniotic sac can rupture, thereby increasing the chance of infection somewhat. Physiologically the top of the uterus is now well above your belly button, and your cervix is descending, thinning out so much it may lead more easily to bleeding or infection, so it's a good preventive measure to keep your vagina very clean.

YEAST INFECTIONS

You should also be aware that some pregnant women develop vaginal yeast infections. According to Dr. Elizabeth Stewart, "Yeast infections may be harder to cure during pregnancy because high hormone levels at this time increase the starch content of vaginal cells, providing good nutrients for yeast. Estrogen also helps yeast attach better to the vaginal cell and then turn into a hypa (stem) form that can cause vaginitis."

It is also possible for newborns to contract thrush (a yeast infection in the mouth) from passing through the birth canals of mothers with yeast infections (oral-genital contact). Don't treat your yeast infection with an over-the-counter product. Check with your obstetrician or midwife first. Common symptoms can include:

- discharge becoming thicker or more odorous
- itchiness in the vagina
- painful urination
- more frequent urination

Condoms Are Not Just for Birth Control

If a woman has a yeast infection or if either she or her partner has a sexually transmitted disease, several medical sources suggest using a condom in the last two months, or even abstaining. This is also recommended for women who know that they contract easily in response to prostaglandins in semen. As you will see in the next chapter, foreplay and intercourse have been documented by some doctors to encourage the onset of labor. And the world-renowned midwife Ina May Gaskin points out that pleasurable intercourse during the last weeks of pregnancy helps the woman's body go into labor because of the presence of prostaglandins in semen. (More on sex inducing labor in Chapter Nine.)

SEXUALLY TRANSMITTED DISEASES (STDS)

There are a couple of STDs that can impact you and your baby. Specifically, herpes and chlamydia are two infections known to be harmful to the baby if passed on during delivery. According to Dr. Glade Curtis, between 20 and 30 percent of sexually active women have been exposed to chlamydia through sexual activity—even oral sex. These infections can go undetected, as they are sometimes symptomless.

As with herpes, the mother exposes the child to chlamydia during delivery as the mucosal tissue of the baby's eyes, nose, and mouth come in contact with the affected tissue when the baby goes through the birth canal. If you have an active infection of either chlamydia or herpes, you may need to have a cesarean. Be aware that condoms as a barrier method are one of the better ways to protect yourself from getting these sorts of infections. If you think you have been exposed to chlamydia but are asymptomatic, rapid diagnostic tests can be performed in your doctor's office to determine exposure. Although you can't use tetracycline to clear it up, erythromycin is an option.

Symptoms of chlamydia:

- burning, itching genital discharge
- painful and frequent urination
- pain in pelvic area

Sore Backs and Swollen Feet

When your little tootsies are sore, your whole life feels bad. One of the best things for the swollen feet and bad backs is gentle manual ministrations from your partner. Not only will it connect you physically, it will give the added benefit of moisturizing your skin and helping your system move some of that increased body fluid away from your feet. Many women also find their feet change size. This is due to the hormone relaxin, which acts on the connective tissue of your body to enable your hips and pelvis to open that additional 20 mm to allow the baby's head through.

Stretch Marks

There are two main factors that will influence the appearance of stretch marks: your inherited skin characteristics and how much weight you gain. As Dr. Jules Black told me, "Whoever comes up with a cure for stretch marks will make billions." Lovely massages from your partner with various lotions may make your dry, overstretched skin feel better, but there is nothing on the market that prevents or repairs them. But keep in mind, some men value these lines of love. As one man shared,

"I know my wife hated her stretch marks, but for me they were like a tattoo. They remind me of how amazing her body was in being able to create our children."

Windy Tales

Ladies, there are a few natural but not exactly sex-inspiring digestion issues that crop up during your third trimester. Your digestion will get slower during this third trimester, which may result in more gas and wind for you. There is slower gastric emptying thanks to the higher levels of progesterone, especially in the third trimester. As a result, there is less gastric acid produced, and the slowdown of your body's ability to digest food can increase production of wind.

Another possible impact to your digestion slowing down thanks to the smooth muscle relaxant effect of progesterone is constipation. And the reason is the longer that stool is maintained in the lower bowel, the more water is absorbed. In turn, the harder and more compact the stool becomes. It's best to make sure you ingest what makes things move for you—including lots of fruits, veggies, other foods that contain fiber, and, of course, liquids.

One woman said she felt like a teenage boy "burping and farting all the time. Will this ever end?" she asked me. The answer is yes. As soon as you deliver, the gas will cease.

Women who regularly eat spicy foods may want to keep the following in mind. There is a natural pain-blocking effect that occurs during labor as the baby's head passes down the birth canal, compressing the hypogastric and pelvic nerve systems. Dr. Whipple's research on nonpregnant women who have a diet very high in hot peppers, whose active ingredient is capsaicin, did not get the natural pain-blocking effect of vaginal self-stimulation that women whose diets had a medium to low level of hot pepper consumption did. This has led to Dr. Whipple's hypothesis that women whose diets contain very high levels of capsaicin will have more painful deliveries than women whose do not. And, anecdotally, women in India are told not to eat spicy food for about three months before they deliver for the same reason.

How Pregnancy Has Contributed to General Science

Some pregnant women find they no longer experience the symptoms of chronic conditions such as arthritis and asthma. Why? In observing how pregnant women often had their arthritis and asthma get better, researchers suspected it was the heightened progesterone and estrogen that were responsible. Not so. It turns out the high levels of sex hormones are accompanied by high levels of corticosteroids produced by the adrenal glands to keep the embryo safe during gestation. You can now thank pregnant women for the breakthrough that the increased levels of corticosteroids are the ticket to alleviating asthma and arthritis.

The Great Debate: Sex or No Sex—That Is the Question

Although the warning list on page 95 still holds for the third trimester, the main concern physicians warn pregnant women about regarding sex during the third trimester is the risk of bringing on premature labor and delivery. Otherwise, most doctors believe that neither intercourse nor orgasm *alone* stimulates uterine contractions, so women with normal pregnancies are given the green light to go for it right up to delivery day. Victoria shared this with me: "My doctor told me you can be doing things until you arrive at the hospital."

Most women, even those who have been experiencing more intense orgasms throughout their pregnancies, have nothing to fear about provoking premature labor. However, if you are feeling short of breath or very clumsy during sex, take care not to overexert yourself. And at all times, whether during sexual activity or your regular pursuits, allow your blood to circulate freely by not wearing anything (clothing or jewelry) that pinches or binds you too tightly.

Warnings to Consider

If you have had a difficult pregnancy, suffer from either pre-eclampsia or an incompetent cervix, have been put on bed rest, or have a history of miscarriages or bleeding, you are likely to be advised by your doctor to abstain for these last few weeks. Again, consult the list on page 95 for more warnings that preclude sex. But remember, you can save your desire for later!

CAN THE BABY FEEL WHAT YOU'RE DOING?

A concern I have heard expressed over and over again is whether the movements associated with penetration bother or even harm the baby at this late stage. One woman told me, "Even though I was up for sex, my husband started to back off. He said entering me just didn't feel right. I assured him it was safe, but he still felt uncomfortable—he thought the baby would be hurt." This is a very common misconception—especially among men. Fortunately, the more information you can give your man about how safely snuggled your baby is in his or her cocoon, the more likely he is to let go of his fear.

One reason for this misconception is that by the third trimester, you can now often feel the baby's reactions to your actions: between weeks twenty-eight and thirty-two, fetal activity becomes more clearly defined. Some women say that when they are busy, their babies seem to go to sleep. Other women say that when they are busy, they can feel their babies move around, stimulated by their own movement. Other women feel their babies react after eating, finding an increase in kicking and stretching. I know a woman who had to eat hot oatmeal every night or her second child would not settle down enough for her to sleep. How did she know this? "Christa would keep me awake with her kicking. Once I was up, I had to make myself something to eat, and I often seemed to crave oatmeal. As soon as I started to eat it, the baby would settle down. At first my husband didn't believe me, but then he could see how the baby would roll gently on her side and go to sleep. By the way, it's four years later and Christa still wants oatmeal every morning!"

But all the experts point out that if you are otherwise healthy (see the risk factors on page 95), then your baby is not negatively affected by sex, including intercourse. In fact, such stimulation of the baby inside the woman's uterus can be beneficial for the baby, acting like a sort of massage.

You may wonder about jostling the baby or even causing tangles in the umbilical cord. First, remember, the baby is cushioned in an amniotic sac that prevents it from being harmed in all but the most serious incidents, such as a car accident or a severe fall. Second, your actions do not relate to the formation of knots in the cord. According to Dr. Curtis, knots in the umbilical cord occur when the baby shifts around and a loop forms through which it then moves. There is nothing the mother can do to cause or prevent this.

Orgasms and Labor

You needn't worry about orgasms inducing labor. As George A. Macones, M.D., associate professor of obstetrics, gynecology, and epidemiology at the University of Pennsylvania, says, "The contractions that you may feel during and just after orgasm are entirely different from the contractions associated with labor."

BLOWING ISN'T SAFE

Do advise your partner to be aware of blowing air into the vagina during oral sex. The bubble can travel through the highly vascularized cervical and uterine tissue to your bloodstream and cause an air embolism, which is extremely dangerous. And as a sex educator, I feel compelled to ask, What could possibly be sexually stimulating about air in the vagina coming out like the vagina passing gas? I assume that blowing air into the vagina must occur by mistake during oral sex. As one woman said, "Why the heck would anyone blow into your vagina? I can't imagine it feels very good!"

N*oisy Orgasms Are Good*

Dr. Jules Black has observed that patients who have very intense, large, noisy orgasms tend to have disproportionately easier and shorter labors.

SEX WHEN THE BABY HAS DROPPED

In the last week or two weeks of your pregnancy, the baby enters the birth canal to prepare for delivery. This is known as lightening, or more commonly, it is said the baby has "dropped." A side benefit to your baby's dropping is that now you will have more room in the upper abdomen, which allows you to breathe more easily. A drawback, however, may be increased pressure on the pelvis, bladder, and rectum or the sensation of pins and needles (tingling or numbness in the pelvic area). For these reasons, you may find that penetration feels different now.

According to Dr. Elizabeth Stewart, this change in sensation may be due to changes in the connective tissue of the vagina preparing for delivery. There is an increase in the size of the muscle fibers, which can stretch the vaginal walls so that sometimes the lower portion of the front wall of the vagina bulges downward slightly. This may cause a tighter feeling for you and your partner. Some women like this tightness (as do their partners), but others say it can feel uncomfortable.

CONTRACTIONS: ORGASM OR LABOR?

The closer you get to your due date, the more you may wonder whether you can tell the difference between contractions from orgasm and those of labor. Of course, an orgasmic contraction tends to be pleasurable, and a labor contraction is painful. Dr. Marc Ganem further elucidates that the orgasmic spasms of a profound orgasm (as opposed to labor) are essentially vaginal and not uterine, which is why orgasmic contractions are not a concern in a normal pregnancy as a way to initiate premature labor.

Yet it is important to keep in mind what your body undergoes as it begins labor so that when you are within days of your due date, you can distinguish between false labor (Braxton Hicks contractions) and the onset of real labor. Again, some women choose to have sex in an attempt to induce labor. But if you do not want to induce labor, it may be helpful for you to keep in mind the three stages of labor.

The first occurs when you experience uterine contractions of great enough intensity to cause thinning (effacement) and dilation of the cervix, so the baby can be pushed out. These contractions will be regular, increasing in frequency and strength. Time them from the beginning of the pain to the end, and try to find a pattern. Before you call your doctor, it is important to time the frequency of the contractions and how long they last. When the cervix is dilated to 10 cm, stage one is complete, and your cervix is big enough to allow the baby's head out.

The second stage of labor begins when the cervix has completely dilated to 10 cm and ends after the baby has been delivered. The third stage is after delivery of the baby, when the placenta and fetal membranes are delivered.

How will you know if you are experiencing false labor or having postorgasmic contractions? Irregular, short contractions under forty-five seconds that occur in your groin, lower abdomen, and back are unlikely to be real labor. Labor-inducing uterine contractions cause pain that starts at the top of the uterus, radiates over the entire uterus, and extends through the lower back to the pelvis. Such pain can also be an indication of back labor.

Slowing Down Labor

If you are at high risk for early delivery, rest assured there are many drugs that can slow down your contractions and even stop them should you go into early labor. Ask your doctor about the types of activities you might want to avoid, such as lying on your back or having sexual intercourse.

As Hot Mamas, we need to be conscious of maintaining the innate power of our femininity, and at no time is the power of the feminine more naturally obvious than in a woman who is about to have a child. May I suggest that you ponder your own femininity as you embrace your big, beautiful body, and get ready to explore in the next chapter the positions and techniques that can enhance your sexual pleasure and that of your partner.

9

Does Size Really Matter?
and Other Ways to Get Creative
in the Bedroom

During the third trimester your sex life is likely going to align with the impact of the final physical changes of your body. The more dramatic these changes are, the less inclined you will be to desire or try certain styles of sex. However, as pointed out in the previous chapter, for most women, sex can continue until you deliver.

The "Does Size Really Matter?" of the chapter title refers to the size of the lady. Specifically, I am referring to two components of size: the mental and the physical. Your mental size is all about how you feel. How comfortable do you feel about your size? In my experience listening to hundreds of women, it's the mental size that determines whether or not a woman taps into her sensuality and desire enough to enjoy sexual pleasure.

Although the size of a woman's abdomen is definitely a factor in making sex comfortable, the breadth of one's belly does not have to preclude sex, including intercourse. The woman who gains twenty-three pounds and looks like she swallowed a basketball often has a very different experience than a woman who gained seventy pounds and feels like a whale. Yet having said that, numerous women who described themselves as huge were sexually active until they went into labor. In other words, they may have felt huge, but they didn't think their size had anything to do with limiting their sexual pleasure. As one woman shared, "My husband simply could not get enough of me during my pregnancy with our son. I was huge—just enormous—and all he could say was, 'Babe, I can't keep my hands off you!'"

The positions most preferred during the final months invariably involve support for the mother's abdomen, back, and hips; reduced motion; and often little to no flexibility of the woman's hips or knees. The bigger the lady gets, the fewer your options. However, like all events in life, when there are fewer things to choose from, you tend to choose with more thought on each option. So whether it is oral sex, manual stimulation, penetrative intercourse, masturbation, or creative cuddling, for many couples lovemaking during this trimester is quieter and more creative.

As I wrote earlier, sex during your third trimester is often about two things: comfort and connection. Whether you and your partner enjoy some of the options described here or find pleasure from merely holding hands in bed, know that if you have remained close throughout the previous nine months, you will no doubt be able to resume your passionate embrace of each other after your child arrives.

Side Support Sex

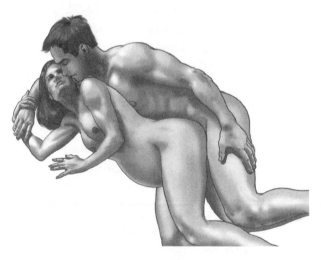

Fig. 27

Figure 27 shows one of the easiest and most gentle styles for sex heading into the final months. The lady is on her left side with a slightly raised leg to allow ease of entry. Either partner can stimulate the clitoris manually or with a novelty. A pillow can easily be used to support her tummy, with another between her legs so she does not have to strain to keep her leg up, allowing him easier access.

Female Superior Position

Those women who prefer Female Superior position find having a support to balance on while using the strength of their legs as in figure 28 allows the lady to control the depth of penetration while placing herself exactly where she prefers.

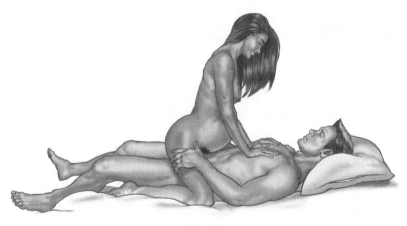

Fig. 28

With her hands on his chest gently stabilizing her, and using the strength of her thighs for motion, there is no pressure on her abdomen and he can watch her abundant breasts as she uses him for her pleasure. You can use pillows to assist your positioning or use the Liberator® Shapes to get you to the right angle.

D*oes It Feel Tighter in There?*

Some women will feel as if there is tightening around their partner's penis, and indeed that is the case. Yet even with the shortened vaginal vault, there is no need for the man to worry about hitting the fetus or the cervix during thrusting, as the head of the penis, the glans, will naturally slip under the neck of the cervix into the area known as the cul-de-sac, the curved innermost end of the vagina. The foreshortening can lead to enhanced pleasure particularly for women who enjoy deep penetrative thrusting. And, again, Dr. Ganem reassures that the act of making love will never result in the penis's touching or hitting the baby.

The Side Angle Approach

The Side Angle approach in figure 29 works well especially for those couples who know there is more sensitivity on one side of the vaginal vault than the other.

At this point in your pregnancy, it is best to lie on your left, so the inferior vena cava does not get compressed by the baby's weight. Chances are, the cushions of your couch will never be looked at the same way again. Here you see the lady's full tummy is easily supported by cushions, and he has easy access to penetrate. An added pleasure is that they can watch themselves—more than likely you may add this position to your postpregnancy repertoire.

The best thrusting for this position tends to be shallower, as the man needs to use her leg and his balance to maintain motion, and too

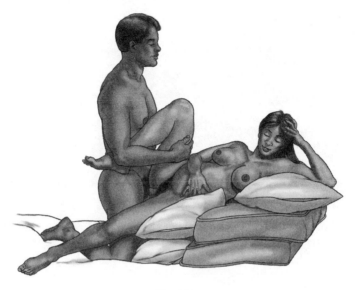

Fig. 29

much motion will result in "fall-out." Should the lady feel inclined, she can easily use her hands to heighten the sensation.

Sidesaddle (aka Le Cheval)

The Sidesaddle in figure 30 is a favorite for those couples who enjoy full lower-body contact. As one woman said, "I loved this position because the friction was so intense—we couldn't really move a lot. And my husband didn't even have to thrust as much as usual. I actually orgasmed from my clitoris being stimulated."

This position with her legs lifted takes the strain off of her lower back, and she can relax into the sensation, as she can rest her legs on her partner's thigh and hip. One woman's comment was "I loved being able to feel his thighs as he thrust into me; he is a runner, and I'd never felt the strength of his legs so intensely." And both partners have their hands free to easily adjust position or stimulate other areas.

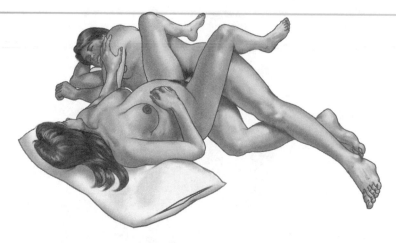

Fig. 30

Rear Entry

This position, with her tummy fully supported by pillows, a cushion, or an ottoman, is many couples' staple for the last three months.

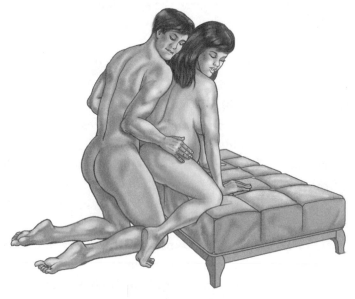

Fig. 31

A variation of Rear Entry can be seen in figure 31, where the woman is in a more upright position. She is elevated above him so she can open her thighs easily for penetration while at the same time feeling stable because of his thighs being curved underneath her. Some women have said this is more comfortable than leaning over more fully in Rear Entry, in which they tend to feel as if they are going to break in two with the weight of the baby.

Manual, Oral, and Other Options

For some couples, her size, her comfort, his concern about her and the baby, all lead to nonpenetrative styles of intimacy. Such couples reported enjoying manual, oral, and self-pleasuring sex.

MANUAL

Manual stimulation either by yourself or by your partner is a standard part of most couples' nonpregnant sexual repertoire. For some pregnant couples "necessity is the mother of invention" in their quest to try new, nonpenetrative options, leading them to expand and/or add new manual ideas for both. "I love going down on him, but I had so much saliva and gagged so easily I simply couldn't after about six months. So I got some great lube and created my own penile massage parlor. I'd lay him out like he'd be at a massage place, and it became part of how I took care of him. And it was part of his fantasy of getting extra services—as he called it, "a rub and a tug."" Be sure to use a nonperfumed, water-based lubricant on him so that if you do decide to go on to penetrative sex, you reduce your possibility of irritation from the product.

ORAL

You may want to try some oral pleasure, as shown in figure 32, where in Sit on My Face (SOMF) she is in control of her clitoris's placement, or as in figure 33, where she is using pillows under her hips to position herself for ease of access while the increased height allows him to keep his neck comfortable.

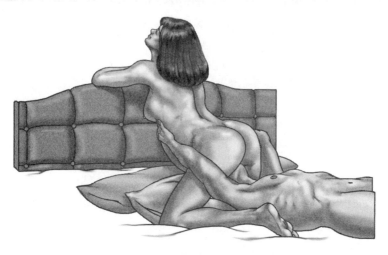

Fig. 32

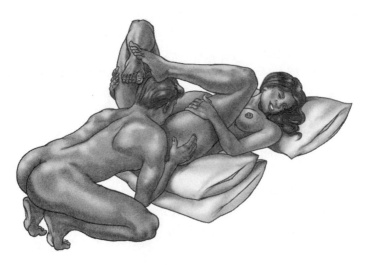

Fig. 33

The beauty of these forms is that they require little or no effort on the part of the woman. She is able to keep herself in her chosen position, so she can completely relax into what her partner is doing.

MASTURBATION, OR SELF-PLEASURING

One of my clients said that by the third trimester, her Braxton Hicks contractions were so common that she felt uncomfortable having intercourse. Did she lose her sex drive? "Not at all," she explained. "I had to masturbate every day—and I have never been a big masturbator!"

Women (and men) enjoy the freedom and exactitude of masturbation. Karoline Bishof, M.D., points out in her brilliant Ph.D. dissertation that there are two types of sexual desire—dyadic (partner-related) and solitary (self-directed). Interestingly, in her long-term analysis of the impact of pregnancy on the sex life of a couple, she points out that "solitary desire appears to be closer to what is termed sexual drive while dyadic desire is a more complex construct." The implication here is that when women continue to connect to their own desire through self-pleasuring, they give their libido a better chance of staying intact—regardless of the challenges of pregnancy. So, ladies, pleasure yourselves away! In the long run, you will be doing yourself . . . and your partner a wonderful service!

Sex to Induce Labor

Many women who go past their due dates look for ways to induce labor. Should you want to induce labor, there is a type of sex that a friend of mine refers to as Roto-Rootering, which may just do the trick. This entails any type of sex that results in a good deposit of semen on the cervix. As one of my clients shared, "At my thirty-eight-week appointment, my doctor said, "OK, you're one centimeter dilated. Time to start getting freaky in the bedroom. Sex to get the baby in, sex to get the baby out!"

There are several factors related to sex that induce labor, including the prostaglandins in the man's semen, the oxytocin released from rubbing the woman's nipples, and the uterine contractions from an orgasm. But a good orgasm close to your delivery date may also work wonders at moving that baby. As one gentleman recalled quite fondly, "My wife and I were in bed knowing this was her 'due date,' and I volunteered to do my manly duty and see if I could get things going. Well, indeed it did—between me and Hitachi Magic Wand my wife went into labor almost immediately."

Prostaglandins in semen are shown to help bring on labor contractions. Dr. Jules Black suggests thinking of their effect in this way: imagine an orchard, and during the growing season the apples are solidly attached by their petioles to the branch so no amount of wind will make them fall off. When the fruit starts to ripen, it can easily be dislodged by the wind. The pregnant cervix is much the same as the apple. It starts out firm in the early stages of pregnancy and then begins to soften and "ripen" right around the time a woman is about to deliver. This ripening usually starts around thirty-eight weeks. When prostaglandins are introduced to this ripened cervix, they can cause it to soften and dilate. And the amount of semen necessary? One to five ml of ejaculate—the normal volume most men ejaculate with one orgasm. Be aware that the prostaglandins used to induce labor are synthetic and are much more concentrated than those that are naturally occurring in men's semen.

Labor can also be induced by the weight of the baby low down in the vagina, which elicits the Ferguson Reflex, a spinal reflex that releases a spurt of oxytocin when the lower vagina is distended, initiating labor. Women who notice an enhancement of their orgasms due to lower vaginal distension are probably experiencing this same Ferguson Reflex.

NIPPLE MASSAGE

Lightly stimulating, rubbing, or massaging the nipples can induce labor. The closer to a woman's due date or beyond, the better this technique will work. This action requires concentration and effort to work. One rubs the nipple and the area surrounding the areola for fifteen minutes, and alternates to the other side for fifteen minutes, for a total of one hour three times a day. This will heighten the production of oxytocin, the hormone that promotes uterine contractions and milk ejection. As one woman shared, "This was my third pregnancy, and it worked like I couldn't believe."

The stimulation of the nipples assists both labor onset and milk flow. When a baby suckles, the milk squirts out and specifically opens the blood vessels in the skin of the breasts, warming them, so there is a lovely heated pillow for the baby's cheek.

Giving Birth Can Be a Sexual Experience

While not in the majority, a few women have reported experiencing orgasms as they deliver. Impossible? *Au contraire,* my friends. Indeed, as the baby comes down the birth canal, his or her head puts pressure on two important nerve systems—the hypogastric and the pelvic—which has an analgesic effect, according to research done by Beverly Whipple et al. Additionally, the intense pressure on those nerves can induce orgasm in some laboring women. Such a response makes sense when you realize that firm stimulation of these two nerve systems is responsible for women's ability to experience G spot, vaginal, and cervical orgasms. As one woman recalled, "My husband was helping me into a warm shower while I was in heavy labor, and all of a sudden I felt this deep orgasm building up inside me. Now, you have to know I wasn't feeling the least bit sexed up at that moment. When I told my husband I'd just had an orgasm, he reminded me of what I'd said the moment I conceived Cleo—that I had had the most amazing-hugely-warm-glowed-inside-me-forever orgasm. I mean, how profound is it to have giving birth be a full-circle sexual experience?"

The connection between sexual pleasure and labor and delivery is even more profound. Dr. Jules Black shows the multifaceted parallel between the two processes in the graph below. Take a look:

Natural Childbirth		Sexual Excitement and Orgasm
During early contractions, breathing becomes deeper. Second stage of labor brings deep breathing with breath holding.	*Breathing*	*During early stages of arousal, breathing becomes faster and deeper. As orgasm approaches, breathing may be interrupted.*

NATURAL CHILDBIRTH		SEXUAL EXCITEMENT AND ORGASM
Tendency to make noise, grunts, especially in second stage of labor.	Vocalization	Tendency to make gasping, sucking noises as orgasm nears.
As birth climax approaches, the face gets an intense, strained look.	Facial Expression	As orgasm approaches, the face gets what Kinsey et al. called a "tortured expression."
The upper segment of the uterus contracts rhythmically.	The Uterus	The upper segment of the uterus contracts rhythmically.
Mucus plug from opening of the cervix loosens.	The Cervix	Cervical secretion may loosen mucus plug, thus opening cervix for sperm.
Contract periodically in second stage of labor; strong urge to bear down develops as delivery approaches.	Abdominal Muscles	Abdominal muscles contract periodically during sexual excitement.
Woman flat on her back, legs bent and wide apart.	Position	Typically, missionary position (woman on her back, legs wide apart).
Woman tends to become uninhibited, particularly as baby descends the vagina.	Central Nervous System	Inhibitions and psychic blocks are relieved and often eliminated as orgasm nears.
Delivery of baby through narrow passage requires unusual strength and body expansion.	Strength and Flexibility	Unusual muscular strength often develops. Many people are able to bend and distort their bodies in ways otherwise not capable of.

NATURAL CHILDBIRTH		SEXUAL EXCITEMENT AND ORGASM
During labor, vulva becomes anesthetized with full dilation so that the woman must be told of the emergence of the baby's head. There is a tendency to become oblivious of surroundings as delivery approaches. Amnesia develops. Suddenly, delivery complete, the woman becomes wide awake.	*Sensory Perception*	*The whole body of the sexually aroused person becomes increasingly insensitive, even to sharp blows. As orgasm approaches, tendency to become oblivious to surroundings. There is a loss of sensory perceptions sometimes leading to moments of unconsciousness. After orgasm, there is a sudden return of sensory acuity.*
After birth there is a flood of joyful emotion, which Dr. Granthy Dick-Read describes as "complete and careless ecstasy."	*Emotional Response*	*After coital orgasm, there is a strong feeling of well-being in most people.*

While you may not be one of the lucky few to experience labor and delivery in quite this pleasurable a way, you can use the sensual and sexual energy between you and your partner to push yourselves into parenthood.

As you cross the great divide into parenthood, I wish you the best of luck. I have supreme confidence that you will not only arrive safely on the other side, with a wonderful baby in your arms, you will also rediscover yourself.

The "Fourth Trimester"

10

Reconnecting with Yourself and Your Partner

THERE ARE ENDLESS BOOKS about infant care. Breast or bottle? Cloth or disposable? Colic or croup? You'll find tomes on weight loss and how to manage your baby's sleep patterns. But short shrift is given to a topic of huge importance to this new phase of your life: how you can reconnect with your lover and yourself after introducing a baby to your life.

But before we get to the subject of how you can help your body heal physically and how you might want to get back in the sexual saddle, so to speak, I feel it's necessary to address just how complicated the postpartum period can be for women, and why three words come to mind: support, validation, and understanding. At no time in your life are you likely going to be more in need of and receive more benefit from these three behaviors than after your relationship has welcomed a baby. Truly, ladies and gentlemen, the reason my clients asked me to look into the impact of pregnancy and a baby's arrival on a couple's sexuality was so they could be aware of the things that can cause and continue the physical distancing between couples. They wanted me, in hard terms, to give them advice on how to avoid the all-too-common slippery slope of no-sex-after-kids. They asked me how their sex life was likely to change, what the snafus to watch out for were, what other couples had to say about this transition into parenthood, and what the medical/therapeutic world had to say. It became blazingly clear that parents wanted to be prepared. These were couples who knew they and they alone were responsible for making their relationship work.

One of the more important messages from women and men who have gone before you is that you should make your priority list and stick to it. If your marriage and your child's health are your priorities, then give yourself permission to do what you need to do and not what you think others think you should do. We all have only twenty-four hours a day to accomplish all that we want to accomplish, and perhaps your pre-motherhood list of priorities needs to be adjusted to fit your new life and its responsibilities. You and you alone know at the end of the day those efforts that resonate with your heart and those that don't.

All that said, I encourage you to approach the "fourth trimester," the one to six months following the birth of your child (or children, as the case may be!), in a spirit of openness and acceptance of where you are. Generalizations never work, but they work even less at this point in your life. So as you contemplate or navigate your transition from pregnant woman to mother, let's see how and when *you* want to return to being a sexual being.

Realigning Yourself with the World

First, to make the most of your life, your partnership, and your new family, you will have to make an effort to balance your responsibilities and to set priorities, and you may consider putting yourself, your partner, and your relationship right near the top of that list. Yes, higher on the list than the vacuuming, that new report due at work, or changing the baby's sheets. This shift begins with making yourself take those five-minute showers to keep you feeling good—inside and out—and ends with you and your lover rollicking in bed. But I don't want to sugarcoat reality: it isn't always easy.

Indeed, as you ready yourself to reenter the world of adults, you will probably find yourself needing to prioritize and make some choices. As one woman, Kathryn, shared, "After my daughter was born, it was the most shocking change in priorities. Nothing prepared me for it. Overnight, my list changed to first, my daughter's health and well-being; second, my marriage and staying connected to my husband; third, work; and fourth, laundry. Before her birth—and even up to the last couple of days before delivering her—work seemed to always come first, then my relationship, and then me."

Many women spoke to me of similar changes in priorities, with most or all of them saying that their new babies took precedence. But I find it very important and interesting that most or all women place their relationships second. Why? Because they seem to know intuitively that the emotional, physical, and spiritual health of everyone—baby, mother, father, family—depends on the couple's being a united front.

A*sking for the Help You Need*

A big part of reconnecting with yourself is being able to ask for help when you really need it. Please, please, please do this. If your family is too far away or unable to be by your side in the first weeks after you give birth, there are many services for new mothers offered in most communities, including:

- **Baby nurses**—While such nurses tend to be expensive, they do take complete care of the new infant. They will wake up with the baby in the middle of the night, bring her to you to nurse (if you have decided to breast-feed), and then put her back down to sleep.
- **Doulas**—Usually women, doulas are mommy helpers who are there to care for the new mother more than the infant. They will do errands, go grocery shopping, help bathe you, and let you sleep.

Additionally:

- **Reach out to friends**—even if you have only time for a phone call. Breaking through the baby barrier and reconnecting with the outside world is very important to keeping your sanity during this very dramatic time.

➤ **Keep your man close**—While there are suggestions throughout this book for keeping your man close, now is the time to really let him know when you need him.

Knowing When You're Ready

There is no doubt that the pressures and stress of bringing a new baby into a household can be so disruptive that for many couples, this will bring to a head sexual issues that hadn't been discussed before or hadn't occurred before. One client said,

"The first three months after Jessie was born were a blur. I had a difficult delivery, she was colicky, and it was winter, so I was locked inside, which made me a basket case. Fortunately I had a very wise mother who warned me about how insidious and damaging having a baby can be to a couple's sex life. She saw through her own experience that all the focus and attention goes to supporting the children and not the couple. She told me things would get better around three or four months. She was right. She said we'd have to talk about the two of us and plan for our sex life— even more than when we were college students living at home and sneaking around to do things. She was right again. Her most helpful advice was that it would get better, that things would change but as a couple we would have an even deeper connection if we could weather the changes and turmoil of our baby's arrival. So even before we knew what we would be dealing with, we talked about the 'what ifs' and 'if this should happen' scenarios that would change our sex life. They didn't all happen, but many did, and because we'd anticipated at least part of what was happening to us as a couple, we changed how and what we called sex. Sometimes when both of us were so sleep deprived we wanted to cry,

falling asleep spooning was the best sex we could have had. When Jessie's sleep schedule settled, the rest of the house did too."

This client's comments point to some of the most common issues couples face right after a baby arrives. During the first three months postpartum, most couples are so exhausted and their schedules are so crazy that the most loving thing they can do for one another is to be supportive. This may mean holding hands, snuggling in bed with your newborn, or simply giving each other some time away from the baby to do whatever—sleep, take a shower, watch television.

The stress of caring for a newborn is not to be minimized, but it can be exacerbated if partners are not connected to each other. As Michelle said of her situation, "Even though Paul promised me he was taking off a couple of weeks after Micah was born, he went back to work after three and a half days. I was too exhausted to be angry—that came later—but I was completely overwhelmed. It wasn't the baby—it was me. I needed him near me, knowing what was happening throughout the day. And, of course, when he came home at night, tired from a day's work, all I wanted to do was throw a pan at him. What I did instead was cry." Michelle captures the near despair that some women experience in the first few weeks postpartum. At the root of this blanket of desperate feelings is the woman's sense that she is all alone. Hundreds of women spoke of the same feeling of isolation. Clare said, "It wasn't rational, but I felt that no one understood how I felt. I felt so alone. The mixture of having to take care of an infant who was completely dependent on me, feeling as if Tom [her husband] had abandoned me, and feeling like I wasn't doing a good enough job was just too much. Finally, things turned around when Tom got the message that I needed him."

There is a stark reality involved in this situation: women by and large still do most of the caretaking of an infant. Out of both biological necessity and an instinctive knowledge that infants want and need their mothers, women take on this responsibility as if it were a mission from God. And it is, to a degree. But my concern, which is echoed by many women with whom I consulted, is that women try their best to reach out to their partners and get them involved—as much for the baby's sake as for their own. Women need their partners—to stay connected, to know their partners are invested in them and the new family, and to feel they care.

Without this supportive alliance in place, many women find it next to impossible to feel remotely inclined to intimacy, including sexual intimacy. As Tamara said quite succinctly, "Until I felt comfortable knowing Greg was there for me, I couldn't even imagine having sex."

You and your mate may well both feel some resentment initially. Perhaps you feel unappreciated as a woman, as though you have lost your old sexy self. Perhaps he feels ignored, and all his pent-up sexual energy has nowhere to go. Don't let this fester. Talk openly and honestly with your man, without complaining. Make sure he understands that if you are not accommodating his desires yet, it's not because you don't love him anymore. And, in turn, listen to him. Allow him to feel validated and important. Men would rather you validate their feelings and show that you are on their "team" than be left in a vacuum, trying to figure out what is going on. In *The Breastfeeding Book,* William and Martha Sears put it this way: "Fathers who feel that they are suffering from an acute lack of sex in the first few weeks after birth but develop the maturity to accept delayed gratification of their needs usually find that their overall relationship with their mate improves." Psychologically, this is very sound advice, as delaying gratification is generally associated with more keen, intense enjoyment of whatever the goal is (in this case, having sex again with their partner!). In talking to many men, I also found this to be true, though men were rarely shy about their natural impatience to get back in that saddle!

Joe captured the challenge of this period in this way: "I didn't want to push Sheila; I wanted to respect her need to recover fully. But when four months had passed, the baby was basically sleeping through the night, and our schedule had begun to settle down, I did say something: 'I need to feel you.' And when I said it in that way, Sheila responded appreciatively."

Being respectful, tactful, gentle, and encouraging is crucial. But, again, women need to remain open and willing, and equally respectful of their partners' feelings.

However, if you are not ready to have intercourse—for either physical or emotional reasons—then you need to respect where you are right now, and so does your partner. There are other ways to reconnect with your partner that can, in the short term, create a wonderful intimacy and sense of harmony between the two of you. The number one way to do this among couples I have worked with is by sharing the care of the baby. This may seem self-evident, and yet I have heard too many stories of women still trying to do this job alone. Here are some of their reasons: they let their husbands sleep so they will feel refreshed for work in the morning; they feel better equipped to care for their infants; they don't trust their partners' ability to administer the same level of care and nurturing to the baby.

Including your partner in child-rearing duties will go a long way to making him feel he is part of the new life you are building. Don't be a martyr and feel resentful. It's a long road you're on, with many turns in the path, and your commitment and openness will keep you on this journey together. As one woman suggested, you may need to give him a nudge. "After Genevieve was born, I thought, OK, he'll do *a* and I'll do *b*. Uh huh—didn't happen. It took a few stormy sessions before we sorted out the dance of taking care of her, and my resentment at having to 'do everything' lessened considerably. The best advice I can give new parents? Just know it will get better. The first six months are insane—especially the first three. And try alternating as many feeding/sleeping/changing shifts as possible."

Keep Laughing

As your body goes through yet more changes in the fourth trimester and you and your partner struggle for normalcy amid the whirlwind of new-parenthood, try to keep your sense of humor intact. One client told me about how even before she got home from the hospital, she burst out laughing. Why?

As her husband helped her into the shower, still bleeding, ooz-ing, and stitched up, with unwashed hair and a face bloated from all the IV fluid, she half-seriously asked him, "So how do I look?" His response? "You've never looked sexier."

The Magic of an Open and Willing Attitude

Couples who have traveled this tumultuous and exciting postpartum road state that knowing things will change is very important to a cou-ple's being able to navigate the stress of this time period. They also say that a willingness to define their sexuality by broader parameters helped them get through this stage. Indeed, an attitude of openness and willingness is key to reconnecting with your partner and resusci-tating your sex life after the birth of a baby.

At all times in our lives any activity starts with the attitude of wanting to try, to explore. Therefore, you must be willing to be inti-mate and sexual with a partner after a baby enters the scene. Couples who wait for their libidos and desire to jump-start their lovemaking of-ten have a long wait. As Joann told me, "Did having sex kind of hurt in the beginning? Of course. But since I expected some mild discom-fort, I was willing to put up with it. It only lasted two or three times, and I so needed to feel close to Paul. I didn't want to lose our connec-tion. And the closer he and I were, the less stressful taking care of the baby felt. I was better able to get that magical feeling of the three of us having created a new family."

As you will read in the next chapter, some women experience more than mild discomfort, and there are remedies for such pain. Indeed, sometimes penetrative sex is the last thing added to couples' post-pregnancy sex lives. But most women who take the time and space to heal well not only begin to reawaken their ability to experience sexual pleasure, they also gain much from a renewed intimacy with their lovers.

Mark and Kathleen are a couple with whom I consulted as they began to get sexually reacquainted with each other. Mark said, "I almost felt like she was a virgin again. I took my time, was really gentle, and spent a lot more time warming her up. She and I were both so grateful to feel that connection that we both began to cry—it was just so intense."

Colleen and Kevin struggled at first to become sexually active. Although Colleen received the green light from her physician (you will find detailed information about physical readiness in the next chapter) after about six weeks, she was reluctant to be touched intimately by her husband. "I felt walled off from him. I just couldn't let my guard down. But Kevin's persistence and his willingness to just be close and rub my back or feet gradually made me feel more comfortable. It was like he had to soften me. The first time we made love was awkward, but we kept trying. Finally, I started to feel like my old self again."

Couples emerge from the long duration of pregnancy and the drama of giving birth at different rates. There is no normal time to resume sexual intimacy. What seems to matter most is that couples are interested in trying to revive their intimate connection. They know that, in the long run, their bond—sensual, sexual, spiritual—is what will keep their family together and most happy. Remember Dr. von Sydow's comment about the effects of parental sexuality on the long-term quality of the marital relationship? She said, "If both partners are sexually active during pregnancy and enjoy it, the relationship is evaluated as better" with regard to tenderness and communication at four months postpartum, and more stable after three years.

Keep an Eye on Your Sensuality

New mothers are often surprised by unexpectedly intense feelings. The bond with the new baby is sometimes so sensually gratifying that without even realizing it the woman focuses her energy on taking care of her baby and away from her partner. She may even be possessive of this deep connection with the child, and resent her partner's trying to steal attention away. Be aware that by attempting to take control of the household and all the baby duties, or sinking blissfully into the breast-feeding mode, a woman may end up shutting out her lover.

One woman recalls the moment when she first became aware of this shift in her attention:

> *"My partner and I always had a passionate connection—even throughout my pregnancy. But once our daughter was born, I be-came submerged in her. I went from breast-feeding to sleeping to washing and bathing her. All my interaction with the baby was so satisfying—and so naturally sensual—that being intimate with my partner wasn't even on my radar. Then suddenly my baby was six months old, and I realized I had barely kissed my partner, much less felt any real desire for him. When I brought it up with him, I could see the look of recognition and relief on his face. He said, 'I thought it was just me.' Seeing how sad I had made him made me realize how easy it had been for me to forget about sex altogether—it was as if my body didn't need it because I was get-ting so much sensual gratification from caring for my baby. But our relationship needed sex, and as soon as my partner and I re-sumed having sex, my body was like, 'Oh, yeah—I remember this!' It felt so good to be held in that way again by the man I love!"*

My point here, ladies: this sublimation of your sensuality can hap-pen very subtly, and you may not be aware of it unless you remind yourself. A simple test? Ask your man. I'm sure he will tell you what you've been missing. Become aware of this subtle yet very powerful shift and redirect the satisfying contact with your newborn into your sexual relationship. Let your partner know that he is a priority: re-member that the reason you became a mother is that you were a part-ner first.

What Women Want Their Men to Know

In the past few years in my sexuality seminars, I was continually asked by women not only to address women's issues about sex during pregnancy but also to find some way to tell men what they need *after* the baby is born. In some ways, the meta-message was attention, attention, and more attention. But when I prompted these women to speak candidly and more specifically about what they wanted their men to know, the following list began to form. Women want their men to

- Reassure us that you are there for us.
- Be willing to take care of the infant—without being asked to do so.
- Compliment us on how well we are doing as new mothers.
- Let us know that we are still attractive—and be specific.
- Show us you understand how hard everything is.
- Don't wait to be asked to do something around the house; just do it.
- Show us you are not just interested in sex but in giving us pleasure.

And ladies, you may want to share this page with your man!

What Men Want You to Know

Men shared an analogous desire: they wanted women to know more precisely how they felt during the postpartum experience. With that in mind, I culled a list of their wishes:

Men want their ladies to

- Understand that they are also sensitive to the stress associated with the new baby.
- Appreciate their fear of being replaced by the baby in the mother's affections.

- Be aware that it is difficult not to be included in the mother-baby relationship so evident in nursing.
- Know that they are still afraid that penetrative sex will hurt their partners.
- Understand their worry about their ability to support the family.
- Know that they need to feel desired by them.

D*id You Know?*

When men hear their newborn babies cry, they often experience an increase in testosterone.

Scheduling Sex

Scheduling may seem like it can kill spontaneity, but it definitely increases your potential for having fun. Face two facts about parenthood: 1) if you don't plan it, it is probably not going to happen; 2) the days of spontaneous sex where and when you want it are probably behind you for now.

But this does not mean you can't be wild or wicked!

Planning spontaneity is not an oxymoron. People often say, "Oh I want more spontaneous sex." I say simply, "OK, then plan for it." You are not alone in the "Plan it?" reaction. Think about it: the majority of what we call spontaneous sex was planned, planned because at some point during these periods you knew you would be intimate because that was your intention—on the weekend, trolling a bar, your date night when single, your holiday vacation time. And there is a large section of the hospitality industry interested in couples like you who plan intimacy—these are the couples featured in the advertisements on balconies in robes with morning coffee. So keeping that in mind, know that parents of a newborn become masterful at timetables. Soon you will have less time available to plan with, but this has to be close to the top of the priority list for you and your partner to maintain your sexual connectedness.

And then there is the mental foreplay. You need to think of sexual encounters not as yet another chore on your never-ending list, but as a reward and something to look forward to.

My client Amy told me about how she got out of this rut: "About four months after our son Sebastian was born, my husband started making noises about getting our sex life back on track. Frankly, I wasn't all that interested—I just felt too tired—but I knew he was right and that we needed to pay attention to it, and each other. So we planned that we would carve out some time to be intimate in the mornings, after I had gotten up to feed the baby and put him back down for his first nap. The day came, I got up, took care of Sebastian for the hour he was awake (while my husband stayed asleep), and as I was walking down the hall to get back into bed with my husband, the thought occurred to me that I was just going from room to room in my house taking care of the men. It felt like a chore! So as soon as I got back to bed, I talked to my husband about this feeling, and he understood completely. Bless him, his response was 'Well, then, how about you just lie back and let me take care of you for a little while?' What a guy!"

Amy simply needed to remember that sex was something she could *enjoy* rather than something she had to *perform*. It was that tiny mental shift that made all the difference between resenting her husband and "responsibility" and relishing her relationship and her innate right to sexual pleasure.

Unless you create time in your schedule, you may find it hard to get in the mood. As I mentioned, the entire hospitality industry targets people who plan sex; why not have that include you? One woman, Kathryn, took matters into her own hands: she planned a one-night romantic rendezvous at an elegant hotel in a nearby city. "I wanted not only to surprise him but to give both of us a chance to get in the mood. The fact is, we love staying home with our baby—we love just watching him throughout an entire evening. But when we indulge in this family time, we don't act like a couple. So even though we didn't exactly have the disposable income for a fancy hotel, I thought that it was well worth the money." When I asked Kathryn how the evening went, she said, "Well, let's just say the hotel package included a three-course dinner at a nearby restaurant. We never made it. When we finally came up for air, we ordered room service!"

Whether you go for an expensive night out or a simple motel getaway, a change in locale can do wonders for getting you out of parent mode and into love mode. In short, you need to either grab opportunities when they present themselves or use your creative ideas to make them happen. This is where quality really counts over quantity. You don't need to wait until your baby is asleep. Let him or her play alone for a little while, looking at a colorful mobile while safely in his crib— after all, isn't this the purpose of monitors? If your child sleeps in your room, explore some other areas in your home that might be fun sites for frolicking.

Set the Stage for Sex

Create a sexy mood instead of waiting for the desire to strike you. Intention is the key: start by seducing your own mind, as your body is not prepared for sex until your mind is. Some couples use their old tried-and-true "flags" to each other to set the mood: the candles lit in the bathroom, the Post-it note on the drawer with a lipstick kiss on it to set the mental stage. Try not to hurry; enjoy yourselves in the warm-up. Do whatever works for the two of you in what one couple calls their sexplay. Take a bath together, drink a little wine, give foot massages and head rubs—do something so the two of you are close enough to baby but far enough away to mentally be partners. This attitude is fundamental to your couple well-being and therefore the well-being of your family.

There's a Baby in My Bed!

Should your baby sleep in your room? Or even in your bed with you? These questions are personal choices, not moral issues, and from the many women I have spoken to, no two families feel the same way about it. There are some important factors to keep in mind, however, when you introduce a sleep pattern that your baby will learn to rely on.

As parents, you will be feeding, changing, bathing, and cuddling with your baby endlessly. In the first few weeks when you are getting used to this new and unpredictable schedule, you may find it easier to have your child in the room with you in a bassinet near your bed so you can reach over for those middle-of-the-night feedings. Other parents find that hearing their baby's every breath, snuffle, and snort provokes anxiety, and they prefer more autonomy.

Some mothers enjoy bringing the baby into their beds for comfort or ease. However, according to *What to Expect the First Year* (Murkoff et al.), 50 percent of co-sleepers between six months and four years old developed sleep problems, as opposed to only 15 percent who slept in their own beds. There are various issues of concern (such as: How do you break the habit once you want your privacy back and your baby can't fall asleep alone?), but for me the most vital one is how this affects intimacy with your partner.

Understandably, most parents will feel uncomfortable having intercourse or indulging in sensuous foreplay with a child in bed with them. This is a major inhibitor—also known as the best form of birth control. To achieve a balanced approach to your new life as a couple with a child, I believe there is merit to carving out *one* place for yourself, a zone sacred to you, where you and your lover can be free to be yourselves and to reconnect with your body's desires. You may still opt to have a family bed, in which you welcome your child or children. But to also function as a couple, you need to establish some boundaries and private time so that you can have sex. Renowned pediatrician and author Dr. William Sears, who admittedly falls into the pro-family-bed camp says this: "Since tiny babies have a limited awareness and understanding of what's going on anyway, lovemaking in the family bed is seldom a problem when your infant is only a few months old. As the baby gets older, parents seldom feel comfortable enjoying lovemaking in the presence of a sleeping child. Couples who have successfully employed the concept of the family bed have discovered that the master bedroom is not the only place for lovemaking and that every room in the house becomes a potential love chamber. . . . Another option is to move the sleeping child into another room."

There are a number of good parenting books that address the pros and cons of co-sleeping. One that offers a particularly clear step-by-step process for moving your child from the parents' bed to his or her own bed is *Sleep: The Brazelton Way* by renowned pediatrician T. Berry Brazelton and Joshua D. Sparrow, M.D.

Co-sleeping is very much a matter of personal choice. But whatever you decide, try to make a joint decision with the sensual and sexual well-being of your relationship in mind.

Yummy Mummy or Harried Harpy?

As you emerge from the cocoon of pregnancy and try to summon the energy to reenter the world at large, I have a challenging question for you: would you rather be a yummy mummy or a harried harpy (the fourth trimester version of a fat-n-frumpy)? If you picture your future, do you see yourself as an attractive, sexually active, fully rounded woman and mother, or do you accept the image of the perpetually tired, grumpy mom who not only doesn't have time to shower but doesn't care either? Of course, if you've just given birth, this vision of yourself as a renewed femme fatale may seem a far way off. However, this is less about having the time to make yourself look perfect than it is about attitude.

The stress of juggling responsibilities—be they about your new baby, your home, your relationship, your job—will certainly mean you have less time at the hairdresser, or for getting your nails done or shaving your legs (though in reality shaving takes only an additional minute or two and makes your legs feel so much better!). In that same vein, you can learn to put the baby down for forty-five seconds and brush your hair, apply a little rouge before heading out the door, and grab black boot-cut leggings instead of oversize sweatpants. There is no denying that such small efforts to make yourself look good pay huge dividends in how you feel about yourself and your sexuality, pre- or post-pregnancy.

As Maris shared, "As soon as I could, I got a new haircut and colored my hair. I felt so much better about myself that I actually forgot for a minute that the baby in the car seat was mine!" Now, I don't mean to suggest that to be a yummy mummy you need to forget your child. By no means. Rather, what hundreds of women have told me is that they felt so much more positive about life in general when they began to take care of themselves again.

As you contemplate the best ways you know to take care of yourself, consider doing what you have always done:

- Get a new haircut.
- Color your hair.
- Buy some attractive clothes you can wear until you are back into your smaller favorites.
- Exercise.

Choosing to be a yummy mummy instead of a harried harpy is less about what you do to make yourself look and feel good and more about the attitude with which you approach your new life as a mom. This attitude is one based on sexual confidence, a belief in the power of sensuality, and the trust in your own ability to make yourself happy. Aren't these the values you ultimately want to impart to your new daughter or son? Confidence, power, and trust? The very first way you can instill them is by modeling them yourself. So go for it, you Hot Mama. Be the yummy mummy and knock his—and everyone's—socks off!

In the next chapter, you will get to know more about the nitty-gritty of physical healing. As with so much of pregnancy, women go through this experience in their own unique ways. And though I make some suggestions on how to revitalize your body and spirit through exercise as you gain more insight into how your body heals from pregnancy, it remains up to you to honor and respect your body.

Let the Healing Begin
Stage Four of Your Changing Body

Y OU MADE IT: this is the beginning of the rest of your life as a mom.

You now have a new baby, and your psychology and physiology will begin to adjust. Over the next few months, your body will shift from baby-producing machine back to regular functioning female and sexual partner. If at first the idea of sex seems daunting, don't despair. Though every woman's healing timeline is different—depending on the nature of the birth experience—your body *will* rejuvenate over time. For some women this takes only six weeks; for other women it takes three months. For still other women full healing can take almost a year.

These discrepancies can be due to the relative difficulty of the pregnancy or the birth process, or the women's physical condition when they began their pregnancies. Regardless, there is only so much control you have over how long it may take your body to heal. It's paramount that you pay attention to your body and respect and honor where it is in terms of healing.

As you discover the renewed physical strength that comes from this healing, you will most likely also enjoy a reawakening of your sexual desires and needs. Again, every woman has her own timeline, and therefore every couple has its own. Some women get back in touch with their libido very soon after reaching the six-week mark (the typical reference point used by physicians), while it takes other women a lot longer. Indeed I have heard numerous women say that it's at the six-month mark when they have returned to themselves. As Carrie said, "I felt like a teenager again—more attractive, more of a woman, and I wanted more attention from my husband."

Though it may take some time, your libido and your potential for sexual pleasure will return. Trust yourself. Trust your connection with your partner. And trust that one of the best things you can ever offer your child is a solid parental relationship, one founded not only on love but on erotic connection.

Physical Healing Takes Time

The effect of labor on women's bodies is not to be underestimated. Women often come home from the hospital expecting to have their bodies immediately revert to "normal" and are surprised that recuperation can take some time. A yoga fanatic girlfriend said, "I was too exhausted to even walk around the block the first two weeks." One client complained, "I felt worse after delivery than before! I still looked four months pregnant, and I was sore as hell on top of it!" Alas, there is no avoiding the reality of childbirth and its toll on you.

Generally, women's bodies take about six full weeks to heal internally and externally. In the week immediately after delivery, women begin to lose a tremendous amount of fluid, including water, blood, and urine. As your body adjusts to its nonpregnant state, you will find yourself urinating more, sweating at night (one woman claimed she soaked the sheets for an entire week), and discharging a lot of blood. Don't be alarmed; such fluid loss is expected.

The bleeding discharge is called *lochia* and comes from the uterus shedding the rest of its lining. It can last up to six weeks after delivery. The color can range from red to pinkish brown and is eventually cream. Do not use tampons or have intercourse during this period of time. If the discharge makes you sore or is itchy or smelly, you should contact your doctor.

During the six weeks or so that it takes for your uterus to return to its original condition—a process called *involution*—you may feel afterpains, or contractions. Many women say that these contractions often accompany nursing. A warm water bottle or gentle massage of the anal and perineal areas may help soothe the soreness.

Hemorrhoids, inflamed vesicles that protrude from and/or line the anus, can still be bothersome during this period. Pushing the baby out sometimes creates painful piles. Treat them as you normally would with a sitz bath (a basin of warm water and Epsom salts), witch hazel wipes, and other methods described in Chapter Five. One woman told me her hemorrhoids were so painfully large in the weeks after giving birth that she sought further medical advice. The doctor winced when he saw them but said they were not severe enough to require surgery. He did recommend that she give herself a sitz bath one to four times a day, which she did religiously. In one week, the hemorrhoids all but disappeared.

You may also feel the need to urinate frequently. If this urge is painful, then it is not diuresis (frequent urination), which happens right after delivery when you are shedding hormonally induced water weight, but *dysuria*. If you experience dysuria, you may have a bladder infection, often caused by the catheters inserted during labor. Your doctor can check your urine for infection. And don't worry about bothering your doctor; there are so many things that are unfamiliar right now, the last thing you need is another "What is this?" stress in your life. Empty your bladder as soon as you feel the urge, and remember to drink lots of fluids.

You will also retain about five pounds of excess fluid in the stomach. Dr. Black explains that most women notice diuresis three days postpartum when the high levels of pregnancy hormones drop, at which point the swelling in their hands and feet disappears. Your uterus remains enlarged for up to six weeks. And, if you are nursing, you may be left with a "pregnancy pot," which is Mother Nature's way of ensuring milk production. Dr. Black says, "The place on the abdominal wall around the umbilicus (belly button) is where the body retains fluid to have it ready to make milk. No amount of exercise will get rid of it; the underlying muscles will just be nicely toned up. Once the mother weans her baby, she will lose the 2–3 kg (5–7 lbs.) of fluid retained for lactation" in her breasts and abdominal wall.

Fast Healers

Some women heal very quickly—both physically and emotionally. If you are such a woman, then you may find a lot of the information in this chapter difficult to relate to. If that's the case, feel free to skip it and head right for the last chapter, where you will find provocative ways to get back in the sexual saddle!

Lack of Desire

And what if you simply have no sexual desire? Many women say that in the months after giving birth, they experience a profound lack of libido. This absence of desire is directly related to the hormonal roller coaster that your body is still undergoing.

First, estrogen, one of your primary sexual hormones, and one often associated positively with sexual desire, is still on the move. Although your estrogen tends to increase during pregnancy, it drops off again—and dramatically—right after labor and delivery. And in the ensuing months, the level of estrogen ebbs and flows in its attempts to regulate and get back to normal. The result is a corresponding decrease in vaginal lubrication; with your delicate, healing vulvo-vaginal tissue, your first forays into lovemaking that include intercourse are often painful or uncomfortable, which is why Hot Mamas keep a preferred lubricant handy.

And if you are nursing, the increased oxytocin and subsequent increase in prolactin further dull most new mothers' libidos. Prolactin is produced as a direct result of milk production and nursing. Although you begin increased production of prolactin during pregnancy, this powerful hormone has a particularly negative effect on your sex drive postpartum, lessening, altering, or quashing it completely. As one woman said, "Oh, please, *no more hormones.*"

Oxytocin, the so-called cuddle hormone, is also released in conjunction with nursing. While oxytocin is nature's way of fostering the mother-infant bond and can certainly help women feel more warm and cuddly toward both their new babies and their partners, it also compromises their sexual responsiveness.

Know that the readjusting hormones can kill desire, and the changes in your body may temporarily reduce the intensity of your sexual response, as can sleeplessness, fear of pain, or fear of getting pregnant again. You should know that this too shall pass and you don't need to conquer the world in one fell swoop. First give yourself time to heal, and then decide when you are ready to embrace intimacy again.

Please, give yourself some room here. Many women I spoke with were quite worried and/or upset by their lack of desire. As one woman said, "After six months, I still felt nothing. I became increasingly sad. I felt so bad—for both me and my husband. I so wanted to connect again—and yet there was nothing." Other women said they feared that they would "never return to the land of the living." And while some women feel this lack or absence of libido more than others, these hormones do adjust and regulate with time.

How long does it take? This, too, varies greatly. Some women reported that it took almost a year. Other women said they felt a renewed sexual desire when their new babies reached six weeks. Others said they gradually regained their libido after weaning their babies. Still other women reported not feeling sexual desire for almost four years after giving birth.

So while there may be no tricks of the trade that can instantly replenish the wondrous feelings of sexual desire, there is something you can do, and again, it has to do with attitude. In the same way a meditative mantra works subliminally to soothe, comfort, and encourage you in all your pursuits, so does a conscious awareness of wanting to feel sexual desire again. As the saying goes, "What you focus on, you will create." One couple perfectly expressed this gentle tango: one year after the birth of their first child, Marla and Sean were becoming more and more acrimonious with each other. As each month passed, Sean was becoming more resentful of and distant from Marla, and Marla was feeling more and more disengaged and remote from Sean. She also felt guilty; she knew the reason that Sean was backing away was her complete lack of interest in sex. "I just kept hoping something in me would wake up. I would literally pray for my libido to return—we had always had such a great sex life. But I couldn't really say anything to Sean. I was embarrassed."

Finally Sean spoke up: "We need to do something." Marla could no longer hide from the obvious. "It wasn't like I wasn't aware of the problem. I just didn't know what to do about it," she explained. "When Sean said we needed help, I could hear the pain in his voice. He was desperate. That's when things started to change." What they did quite simply was put the subject on the table and talk about what they wanted in their relationship: they both wanted to keep their connection—especially their sexual connection. They knew that this aspect of their relationship was a huge foundation of the health of their new family. As soon as they opened up the subject, and got in touch with what they wanted to happen, they felt better about each other. Now, Marla didn't see her libido surge overnight. This is reality, not a fairy tale. But she didn't wait for it to descend upon her like some gift from heaven. Instead, she worked at getting herself in the mood by paying attention to the more subtle yet simple ways in which she would prepare herself for a sexual encounter (taking a bath, wearing sexy lingerie, lighting candles in the bedroom). She also relaxed and let herself off the hook. Sean, for his part, was more considerate of Marla as well, taking more time to help her relax. Within a couple of months, their sex life had changed significantly from no sex to sex once or twice a week.

If you accept diminished desire as a new state of being, and being sexual is important for you, your partner will suffer, and so will you in the long run. It's a matter of giving yourself room to respect and honor where you are *now* while at the same time keeping your view on where you would like to be in the *future*.

C-*Sections and Sex*

Women who deliver by cesarean section tend to resume intercourse somewhat sooner than women who deliver vaginally, according to Dr. von Sydow's metacontent analysis of 59 studies of sexuality during pregnancy and after childbirth.

Feeling All Used Up:
The Nap Rule

Too tired to shake the negative attitude? You may be anxious or distracted, bored of lonely. We all know that being tired—OK, being exhausted—is one or the biggest dampers on libido. The time your baby is born can affect his or her sleep cycle, so a baby born at three A.M. may tend to wake up more during the night, whereas a baby born at three P.M. may adapt to night sleeping more easily or sooner. Dr. Jules Black points out an anecdotal correspondence between the time a baby is created (conceived) and the time the baby is born. One couple who both work at the Sydney Opera House knew why their baby was born at five A.M.: that was the time they usually made love. So the bottom line is: you have no control over the new sleep patterns of your household, but you *can* adapt to them.

When Baby naps, so should you. Don't ignore this advice! Napping is the best foreplay you can imagine. However, if the baby doesn't sleep, you need to rely on your partner or caregiver to help you get the sleep you need to heal.

But I would be remiss if I didn't point out the obvious challenge of fatigue to your returning to your sex life. Although the first six weeks of your baby's life do pass in a blur for most women, sleep deprivation can continue to be a problem, and one that definitely impacts your sex life and desire factor. One woman admitted that for the first twelve months of her baby's life, she could not go near her bed—otherwise, she would simply crawl in and go to sleep. Her advice? "My husband and I started sex on the couch. We got in the mood by watching an erotic video together, looking at some sensual imagery in a magazine, or just starting a little manual foreplay. There was something about the slightly public atmosphere of the couch in the living room that spurred us on."

Feeling Stretched Out and Other Aftereffects

The exact changes in a woman's vagina immediately after childbirth have not been well studied, though most new moms can sense a difference, usually describing this as feeling "stretched out." In general, this stretched-out feeling is because the vaginal canal is wider, but it will usually gradually shrink back over the next six to twelve weeks. However, it may not return to pre-pregnancy dimensions. The extent of these changes depends on a number of factors: how large your baby was at birth, how long you pushed for, heredity, and your skin's natural tissue elasticity and strength. In essence, Dr. Elizabeth Stewart says that no matter how elastic your tissue, the vulva and the vagina will never quite be the same after childbirth. The perineum will likely have a scar either from an episiotomy (see page 188) or from the tissue tearing during delivery, which may also make it slightly shorter.

The first few weeks after birth are a time to focus on managing any pain you may experience and healing. Again, warm sitz baths for fifteen minutes a few times daily provide great relief. (You can get convenient tubs from your hospital, your doctor, or the pharmacy.) Do not use oil or scented bubbles in the water. For all intents and purposes, you have open surgical wounds, and they need to heal, so use only water unless instructed otherwise by your caregiver. Anything else may introduce bacteria or be irritating, and that is the last thing you need right now. Gently applying maxi pads soaked with witch hazel and then frozen, Tucks wipes, Dermoplast spray, or aloe lotion to the perineal area will alleviate pain. For relief, some women I know have sat on a Ziploc or full bag of frozen peas or squeezed a sports freezer bag between their thighs, as close to the genitals as they could take it. If it is too cold for direct skin contact, consider wrapping the bag in a dish cloth.

If you've had an episiotomy, you are bound to feel tightness or some pain for the first few weeks as your stitches heal. Avoid infection by wiping from front to back after using the bathroom, having a good hygiene policy at all times, and by spritzing warm water on your rectum after bowel movements. Some women bring a small squirt bottle filled with warm water into the bathroom to make this simpler.

If you have had a cesarean or fourth-degree lacerations, your healing will be slower. A cesarean is major abdominal surgery, and it may take six months or more for the incision to fully heal. You may also feel numbness or itchiness in that area until the nerves regenerate in six to nine months. As Kathy said, "I tore all the way through, and my doctor told me it would be six months before I could have painless sex again. I cried—that seemed an unbearably long time. But my husband was patient and helped me understand we had a lifetime of sex ahead of us. And after ten weeks I felt well enough to try—tentatively—and it was tender but wonderful!"

Another woman said, "After birth there wasn't a lot of sexual gratification going on for either of us. But after about six weeks, we gave it a try and went straight to intercourse—it was painful for me, but a relief to be really close again."

Also, many doctors recommend that you not take baths for at least one month after a cesarean or vaginal delivery, or until your stitches or surgical clips are absorbed or removed, and fully healed. But you can always ask your personal caregiver for her or his advice.

D*o Episiotomies Help or Hinder?*

An episiotomy is a surgical cut to enlarge the vaginal opening, performed routinely by many doctors to avoid jagged tearing of the perineum during labor and delivery. Many women who have episiotomies do not develop any of the procedure's possible complications, such as increased blood loss, infection, abscess, and increased pain. One woman, when I asked her if the stitches were uncomfortable, said this to me: "I couldn't even feel them. My hemorrhoids were so big and painful, they were all I could feel or think about." Her scar healed fine, she had no trouble breast-feeding, and she lost no sensation during sex. And Dr. Black says that he has had women request an episiotomy because their sexual arousal and ability to orgasm had been reduced by the overstretching of a previous pregnancy.

Countdown to Sex

How will you know when you can go for it? Most doctors advise waiting until after your six-week checkup before having intercourse. This is a cautious approach to ensure that you won't tear again or introduce germs to an area that has not yet fully healed. Postpartum there is a spike in the bacteria that can cause disease. Yet why there is this dramatic change in the bacterial contents of the vagina is not known. This is likely the reason for "childbed fever," which killed so many women before antibiotics were available. Factors that may contribute to this are the stress and trauma of the delivery; the delivery of the lochia (normal postpartum uterine discharge); the sudden drop in hormones; and contamination in the vagina from bacteria in the intestines, which may occur with a bad tear. Also the cervix is still open and vulnerable to bacteria being introduced into the uterus during this six-week period. At the six-week postpartum checkup in normal deliveries the cervical canal has returned to its pre-pregnancy size, and sexual activity can resume. Indeed, one day after a vaginal delivery, the uterus shrinks in half. Here's an extra benefit of sex, ladies: hormones released during intercourse can cause contractions that also help the uterus return to its normal state, so sex can actually help flatten your tummy.

Some women feel whole and raring to go before this—my advice is to listen to your body. You should no longer be bleeding, and though you may still feel sore you should not be in great pain. Regardless of the degree of pain, many couples choose to return to sex gradually—beginning with a lot of cuddling, touching, and manual stimulation (you will find specific suggestions and tips in the next chapter). Other couples are anxious to have intercourse.

Experiencing some pain the first few times you have intercourse after birth is normal. Some of this pain can be alleviated with lubrication (one reason you are less moist than usual is the low estrogen levels, and dryness is worse if you're breast-feeding). Things will need to be slower and more gentle, and having both of you very well lubricated will ease penetration. Erika said, "After my fourth child, it was like there was a sore on the inside that I had never had before, and without the lubricants Lou recommended, sex would have been too much. The sore eventually shrank, but we continued to use the lubricants because it made our sex life seem more spontaneous. I was ready faster and wasn't worried about it hurting." Slippery Stuff and Intimate Moisture (by Very Private) are both good water-based lubricants to use.

Although for many men there is no feeling in the world that compares with entering their partner's vagina, nowhere is it written that just because he has entered you does he have to stay there to orgasm. One solution came from one Catholic couple who practiced the rhythm method of contraception. "We were used to having to have him pull out and use oral or manual to continue our pleasure. So after Derek was born, we used a modified style for my husband to enter me for a few minutes. I have always just loved how he fills me up. Yet after my episiotomy, I was so tight that the only sensation I could deal with was him being inside and staying still. It was as if the skin had to get used to it all over again. And nothing, absolutely *nothing* would have happened if we hadn't used lubricant." Perhaps you can follow the lead of those who practice this style of rhythm method and create your own style until you are ready for and comfortable with the full-penetration thrusting through to orgasm. For some couples, this may take months.

But as one woman said, "After five months the pain was still so intense, all I could handle was my husband just being inside me. He couldn't move. Then after, I would ask him to withdraw and I would pleasure him in other ways." A pain as persistent and profound as this is called dyspareunia, or pain with intercourse. As another woman described, "I had this searing pain on one side of my vagina after the birth of my fourth child. My OB said it was scar tissue and that after a while the pain should subside. She gave me a standard water-based lube, but it wasn't enough. It wasn't until I got the most lubey lube [that] sex was at all comfortable for me."

Birth Control Is Still an Issue

Contrary to what you may have heard, ovulation can occur at any time after birth, even when breast-feeding, so be sure to think about birth control once you resume sexual activity if another pregnancy is not planned. Post-delivery, my younger sister got pregnant one of the first times she and her husband had sex—four months after her second son was born. Her two sons are thirteen months apart. Be aware that while low-dose oral contraceptives suppress ovulation, estrogen can also inhibit breast milk production. Barrier contraception such as the diaphragm, the cervical cap, the vaginal sponge, the condom, or spermicide foam may be a better bet if you are nursing. Also, you want to choose something that is kind to your vaginal tissues and not irritating. An IUD can be discussed during your six-week checkup.

News Flash

You *can* get pregnant if you are nursing.

You *can* get pregnant if your periods have not yet resumed.

You should use contraception whenever you have intercourse!

Is Surgery the Answer to Stretching and Other Post-Delivery Conditions?

Some women with whom I have spoken are very bothered and distracted by the "stretched-out" feeling they have after childbirth. As one woman put it, "I couldn't even feel my husband when he entered me. It was like I had become an enormous well—there was no traction." As I mention above, most women's tissue rebounds in a few months after delivery. However, for some women, no matter how many Kegels they do, their pelvic floor muscles (which give your vagina and uterus their tightness) do not become tighter. In some cases, this lack of tautness is due to the stress and tears of childbirth, which can injure the connective tissue that supports the pelvic floor muscles. In other cases, it's related to genetic inheritance or constant straining. Even women who never have children can experience this stretching in the pelvic floor, due to constant strain from long-term exposure to activities such as intense jumping or heavy lifting. Related to this lack of tightness in the pelvic floor muscles are two other conditions: urinary incontinence and pelvic organ prolapse, in which the reproductive organs literally drop down. Again, Kegels can help these problems if you do them correctly and consistently. If they don't work, then you may want to consult your ob-gyn for a specialist's advice.

Surgery Can Create Pain

Ladies, please be aware that non–medically necessary pelvic floor surgery can actually lead to dyspareunia, or pain with intercourse, which is why specialists such as urogynecologists only do such surgery if there is a very real need for correction.

Worry not. If indeed there has been such serious trauma, there are medical specialists called urogynecologists who will know the surgical procedures that will tighten up the vaginal opening as well as correct prolapsed tissues. In general, this surgery addresses problems with the pelvic floor (it's often referred to as pelvic floor surgery). However, most physicians will not do these procedures until you have completed having children. And Dr. Jules Black suggests that for a nonsurgical approach, women seek out a physical therapist who specializes in pelvic floor therapy. Consult your ob-gyn for recommendations and referrals.

For those of you who wish to tighten up, there are some nonsurgical techniques that may help:

- **Muscle stimulation**—Myoelectric (*myo* means "muscle") stimulation uses small painless electronic impulses to create muscle contractions, exercising the muscle area. Every muscle contraction is naturally an electronic (+ / –) event, so this therapy assists the muscles until they have the strength to do the work on their own.
- **Physical therapy**—The better your posture and pelvic strength are, the better all the operational parts will work. The practice of Pilates can help.
- **Kegel exercises and products to enhance their efficacy**—See page 20.

- **Other vaginal exercises**, such as hip rolls that are used by dancers—check out any basketball halftime show or BET video for illustrations.
- **Middle Eastern dancing** (aka belly dancing)—This kind of exercise is also an option, as it was created to strengthen women's pelvic regions during pregnancy and childbirth.

If you are interested in more nonsurgical techniques to strengthen and tone this area, consult your health care provider for more information.

Ladies, Beware of Cosmetic Genital Surgery

Please be aware there are so-called professionals out there with oodles of degrees who are preying on women's insecurities about their genitals. Offering surgical enhancements, they are merely using genital shots from adult material, which are completely digitally retouched themselves, as the visual templates to surgically modify women's genitals without taking the sexual function and sensation into consideration.

Feeling Blue or Suffering Postpartum Depression? There Is a Difference

You may be feeling joyful, thrilled, and full of energy. But it is not unusual to feel overwhelmed, exhausted, and afraid. You are still on the hormone roller coaster. According to several studies referred to in Dr. Glade Curtis's book, up to 70 percent of new mothers experience postpartum blues to a certain degree. Usually this downer occurs after the first week or two and doesn't last more than one month to six weeks. You may experience a range of symptoms and emotions: anger (at yourself/baby/other kids); loneliness; inability to cope; headache and confusion; mood changes; sleeplessness and forgetfulness. You need to be kind to yourself. Ask for help! Find a support network of friends or other mothers. Take some "me time" to clear your head.

Postpartum depression, on the other hand, is not quite as easy to solve. Some studies indicate that about 15 percent of women experience mild to severe depression after birth (again, this figure is presented by Dr. Curtis, who refers to several studies). If you have personal or family history of depression, have a very stressful life at home or work, are an older mother, or don't have the father's support, you may be at higher risk.

Some doctors believe this depression is related to falling hormone levels, as occur before your menses, and treat it with extra progesterone or estrogen. Dr. Gil Mileikowsky points out that postpartum depression is like hyperconcentrated PMS. Yet the resulting chemical imbalance can cause a serious psychiatric problem that requires hospitalization or medication.

One woman spoke to me about how "sneaky" her postpartum depression was. "I am not prone to depression, but I am rather on the anxious side. After three months, I was so anxious that I was having trouble breast-feeding my daughter, I couldn't sleep even when I was exhausted, and I didn't have an appetite. When I mentioned this to a friend who happens to be a psychiatrist, he put me on a low dose of Zoloft, which does not interfere with nursing or breast milk. Within three and a half days, I was feeling so much better—it was a miracle. Since this happened to me, I tell all my friends who get pregnant." This woman touches upon how difficult it can be to isolate what's happening. Your whole life has changed, your main concern is your new infant, and you expect to be sleep deprived. Sometimes you may not recognize the signs of postpartum depression until they are creating serious problems.

There is no longer a stigma attached to needing psychological help: be sure to check with your doctor about how to handle this situation. You may need to go on antidepressants, but be aware that your ability to take medications will depend on whether or not you are breast-feeding your child.

W*arning Signs of Postpartum Depression*

- Sleep disturbance (even when exhausted)
- Change in eating habits
- Lack of bonding with baby
- Prolonged or unusual fatigue
- Loss of interest in normal activities
- Severe mood swings
- Hallucinations; thoughts of harming baby or yourself

Breasts: Feeding Machines or Erotic Playthings?

Before pregnancy and birth, your breasts were a source of pleasure, not purpose. But if you are breast-feeding, your breasts are no longer exclusively sexual playthings: they are the main nutritional source for your baby. While some women find breast-feeding to be an experience of being at the infant's beck and call, and the voluptuous size of their breasts makes their breasts seem like alien beings, other women find breast-feeding an enormously erotic experience. Indeed, a number of women say that they experience sensual if not sexual pleasure (sometimes to the point of orgasm) while nursing.

The erotic nature of breast-feeding is substantiated further in Dr. von Sydow's study, which showed that "one-third to one-half of the mothers feel that breast-feeding is an erotic experience ('an incredible physical lust')" that sometimes leads to orgasm. But interestingly, many of these women also expressed guilt feelings related to their sexual excitement and stopped nursing for this reason.

Regardless of whether you experience your nursing breasts as pleasurable or painful, they are certainly different entities than before. The glands look, feel, and react differently than ever before. When your milk comes in, your breasts will swell and be extremely tender (this will abate once your milk production evens out). To alleviate any pain, you can decompress the buildup of milk pressure using several methods: taking a hot shower, applying an ice pack, or lining your bra with two frozen cabbage leaves (one for each breast). This last piece of advice is from a friend's European grandmother. Apparently, a cabbage leaf is often a perfect fit for lining the inside of a woman's nursing bra, and when it is frozen, it gives women comfort, relief, and support.

Your breasts will remain quite large, as milk is stored in the alveoli. At the cry of your baby, you may *feel* milk rush to your nipples. And when you are aroused, you may even spray milk.

Because of the hormones connected with nursing, non-nursing mothers are often interested in sex earlier than nursing mothers. Oxytocin, which enables milk production, is associated with the lessening of sexual desire. However, nursing mothers can still experience sexual pleasure. You may, however, find your breasts will leak during sex play. This can be rather surprising the first time it happens. In the future, you may want to keep a towel handy or wear a comfortable support bra with nipple pads. You could also try nursing just before making love. If your partner enjoys sucking your breasts, you need not be worried about germs or his stealing milk from the baby—there is plenty more available, as the more your breasts are stimulated, the more milk they will produce. But again, some women don't like extra breast stimulation: accept this and move on to another part of your body that can benefit from some loving attention.

Your nipples may dry out and become cracked or painful. Use lanolin (Lansinoh is a highly recommended product for nipples) to soften them until you become accustomed to breast-feeding. In his classic book, *The Complete Book of Breastfeeding,* Dr. Marvin S. Eiger suggests using a warm compress before feeding and a cold compress after feeding to relieve engorgement. "The warm compresses aid the letdown reflex, and the cold packs relieve swelling and pain." Keeping your nipples clean (Dr. Eiger suggests gently washing your nipple openings "after each nursing with a piece of cotton saturated with warm water") and dry (change your nursing bra and nipple shields frequently) also helps to prevent both clogged nipples and infection (mastitis). Ladies, please feel reassured that any help or questions you may have regarding your desire to nurse can be addressed by lactation consultants. Such specialists are generally provided through the hospital or birthing center where you plan to deliver.

If you are nursing and suffering postpartum depression, you must check with your doctor before taking medication. According to Philip Anderson, a pharmacist and the director of the Drug Information Services at the University of California San Diego Medical Center, no drug for depression is known to be entirely safe for breast-feeding mothers. Certain drugs such as Celexa, Sinequan, Prozac, Serafem, and Effexor, while they may get into the milk, may be safe in small doses. And Zoloft and Pamelor are also acceptable in small doses. If you have further questions, I suggest consulting *Medications and Mothers' Milk* 10th edition (2002) or a psychopharmacologist in your area.

Pumping and Dumping

Most experts agree that having a glass of wine or a beer once or twice a week will not harm either your ability to breast-feed or your new baby. However, as Dr. Jules Black points out, drinking too much alcohol ("more than one standard drink a day per 10kg—or 22 lb.—of body weight) may inhibit the milk letdown reflex, and drinking two drinks a day per 10 kg—or 22 lb.—of body weight may block the reflex completely." If you decide to drink a very moderate amount of alcohol, one client recommends "pumping and dumping" in the two to three hours after drinking any alcohol. Pumping and dumping entails using a breast pump to deplete your milk supply, and then literally dumping it. The same is true if you want to protect against your new baby's absorption of antidepressant medications such as Zoloft. Otherwise safe for mother and baby, if you pump and dump at seven to eight hours after you take your medication, you avoid peak absorption by your child.

Losing the Baby Weight: Where's the Old Me?

It's been a number of weeks, and the pounds are coming off slowly. What's with the round tummy? Why are you always hungry and tired? Do you need to start running marathons to lose this flab? And what if you've decided to nurse? Is exercise even possible? I remember Princess Grace saying that while a woman nurses, the baby's health is the mother's most important focus, and her body will have to be a secondary concern. And although I appreciate much of the princess's wisdom, many women (especially Hot Mamas) can find a way to do both: get exercise while nursing.

Some women make resuming exercise and getting back in shape seem effortless. Sarah Jessica Parker was quoted, after being asked how she got back into such fabulous shape so soon after having a baby (she was stick thin about six weeks after giving birth), as saying more or less, "I'm very fortunate. I have a yoga instructor come to my house every morning while my babysitter watches my son for two hours. Most women don't have that luxury" (this isn't an exact quote but close).

This is all fine and good, but how does the average woman, who has to care for her new infant, take care of a household, and work, make time to exercise? Needless to say, having gorgeous, sexy pregnant celebrities and celeb moms on the cover of *People* magazine is a great thing for pregnant women, but at the same time their appearance does create even more pressure for most women—especially as they struggle to re-find their pre-pregnancy bodies. So how do you figure out how to continue being your gorgeous, Hot Mama self when you tend to feel overwhelmed and exhausted and don't have a staff? And what is realistic? How can you be a Hot Mama on your own terms?

According to Health Canada, up to one-third of mothers are still nine to eleven pounds heavier than their pre-pregnancy weight one year after birth. It's the rare woman who shrinks back to her old size and regains her elasticity without at least some effort. The truth of the matter is it takes willpower and time to find your old self. But you can turn this challenge into something positive. As we all know, a healthy and strong body is a precursor to a healthy and strong sex life!

Whereas most health care professionals suggest waiting until you have stopped bleeding and no longer feel acute pain from stitches before exercising, there are gentle exercises that you can do, which will help the blood circulate in the tender zone between your legs. Some of these exercises can be started almost immediately.

Kegels are more important than ever now, as they will strengthen the pelvic floor muscles and greatly improve sex (as well as urinary continence). And keep in mind, there is data-based evidence of a direct correlation between orgasmic enjoyment and sensation and the strength of the pubococcygeus (PC) muscle: this is the muscle that starts contractions during orgasm, and the stronger the muscle, the stronger the orgasmic sensation.

You can also resume your Kegels while you're still in the hospital. Begin with just five a day at first and then build up your strength. For women who had long durations of pushing and/or a very large baby, the muscle tissue of the pelvic floor is probably going to take longer to get back into shape if it has been grossly stretched.

One particularly exemplary video series, *Better Sex Through Yoga* (volumes 1–3), with Jacquie Noelle, offers very strong recommendations for strengthening your pelvic core and thereby strengthening your ability to give and receive sexual pleasure. The programs are specifically designed for both men and women and combine yoga postures, Pilates exercises, and modern dance for enhanced sexual benefits.

Here are some other postpartum exercise options for new moms:

- yoga
- Pilates

➤ tummy-targeting obliques, by doing the bicycle exercise, sit-ups with legs bent

➤ mild aerobic work, including walking, jogging, and using the StairMaster

➤ strength training with light weights (both yoga and Pilates contribute to strength training, as they use resistance against your own body weight)

Resuming some form of exercise will help you regain not only your shape but your energy and enthusiasm, too. One woman shared her secret: "Walking in the evening with the baby's pram gave me three hugely important things: an exercise walk around the neighborhood made normal by our wacky terrier chasing sticks, time for my husband and me to be together as a couple, and a way to help our son fall asleep."

A new and very popular way for new moms to get back in shape is through Mommy and Baby yoga classes. Such classes are growing in their availability in communities nationwide, as women are finding them to be a great, gentle way to strengthen and tone their own bodies, connect physically and emotionally with their newborns, and learn hands-on techniques for calming, quieting, and relaxing their babies through specially designed yoga moves.

Are you worried that your body will never be the same again? Consider tips from these women who say they are happier with their bodies after giving birth than before:

➤ "I did gentle yoga starting when my infant was about six weeks. I followed a couple of tapes that lasted only twenty minutes, but the results were amazing. I started to feel toned and more energetic in weeks."

> ▶ "I loved to take my new baby for walks and used this time to get my legs back in shape. I couldn't walk very fast, but it didn't matter. The stronger my legs felt, the more in touch with my body I felt."
>
> ▶ "I had a C-section, so I felt kind of weak, especially around my middle. But once my baby was about three months, I started to lift light weights. I didn't really think about my legs and just concentrated on my arms. The more toned they became, the better I felt about myself."

The Ultimate Breast Massage

One of my clients swears by this technique for toning and shaping her breasts—before, during, and after pregnancy. "I learned about this move from a woman who has perfectly shaped breasts, even after nursing three babies. I did it religiously each time after I showered, and my breasts not only held their shape after breast-feeding my daughter for eight and a half months, they also went back to their same size." I have researched this particular exercise and found further support for its benefits in your fourth trimester. Dr. Stephen T. Chang, the author of *The Tao of Sexology,* includes breast massage in his Deer Exercise for women. I have adapted his exercise for our purposes here:

1. Gently rub your breasts (around the nipple) in outward, circular motions. Your right hand on your right breast will turn counterclockwise; your left on your left breast, clockwise.

2. Make these circular motions on the breast (without touching the nipples) for a minimum of 36 times per day and a maximum of 360 times per day.

Dr. Chang points out that one of the purposes of this exercise is to stop menstruation. "When the Deer Exercise is performed, the body reacts just as if a baby were regularly sucking on the breast; the body rushes blood to the breasts rather than the uterus (however, be reminded that nursing by itself is not a foolproof method of contraception). Taoists refer to this phenomenon as 'turning back the blood' because it reenergizes the entire body, especially the sexual organs." He goes on to say that "women should not perform the [complete] Deer during pregnancy. The energy generated by the exercise combined with the accompanying increased stimulation of the sexual glands might induce premature labor."

In the next chapter, you will begin to reap the benefits of your healing process as you take steps to get back in the saddle with your man during what we call the fourth trimester, the one to six months after your baby arrives. Again, feeling ready is individual, and it depends on your being and staying in touch with your body and your heart, and what they both need.

12

Getting Back in the Saddle

IT IS IRONIC that many women, so proud of their size and their tummy's shape during their final months of pregnancy, become self-conscious and sad about how their skin and body have been changed because of giving birth.

I was at a woman's house, and she was lamenting her birth marks from her son. Let me set the stage: that night her household was buzzing preparing for the first major dinner date with the new man in her life, who would later become her husband.

She commented, "Oh, if things continue, he is going to see the stretch marks and go, 'Good God.'"

I asked her one question: "What do you love more than anything in this world?"

Her immediate response: "My son." (Her new man was not the child's father.)

I said, "Those marks are the result of your producing his life. They are part of what brought him here for you. How can that be bad?"

She was silent. At that moment, I could see in her eyes that her stretch marks had new meaning for her.

I know men for whom stretch marks are major turn-ons, as they represent just that, a woman who has brought life into the world.

Many women have shared that their size post-delivery and how they feel about their bodies were major influences on what sexual position they felt comfortable in, and how soon they were willing to try more revealing positions. One mother of two preteens stated, "No one has seen my stomach since the birth of my first child." Such ladies who are shy about their bodies may want to consider some comforting techniques, such as having lovely darkened bedrooms and strategically placed blankets, and wearing cami tops. Some ladies will choose the position that best highlights their best body part. If you know you have great gams, make sure they are a focus of play, such as in the rear entry position of figure 34. In this position, the woman can rest her upper torso on the edge of the bed supported by her arms, and have her legs be his main focus—well, OK, part of the focus. If you are concerned about a still-loose tummy, choose a position in which gravity performs its slimming move.

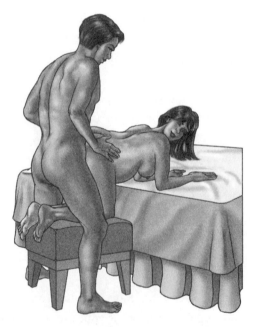

Fig. 34

Whatever your choices may be, make them yours and yours alone; do not feel pressured. Some women cannot wait to have penetrative intercourse after delivery; for others that is hardly the case. For other women who are more uninhibited and therefore more comfortable with their postpartum shape, the world is their oyster. Below I describe some of the positions that are most appealing to women (and their men) in the period following giving birth.

The Scissors Position

Also known as the X position, figure 35 presents a postpregnancy favorite. There are a number of reasons for this: 1) you can adjust so there is no weight on her stomach, which may still be sensitive; 2) the lady's back or hips may be sore; 3) the man can enter at a different angle, which may be preferred due to a newly healed episiotomy scar that is too sensitive or a side of the vagina that is tender; 4) the gentleman may prefer a position that allows thrusting but isn't as strongly stimulating so he will last longer; 5) they may both want to stay connected after the act, and this allows them to rest or fall asleep should they choose; 6) there is less profile in the bed if they don't want their child to see.

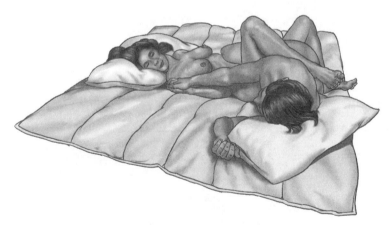

Fig. 35

Semireclined Position

This is another position in which the couple has very good control over the angle of penetration. In this position the man can angle himself to avoid the cervix, which may still be sensitive, as well as any sensitive healing area, as he is not using the standard north-south direction.

This is a favorite not only for after pregnancy but during the late stages of pregnancy, as the woman's back is nicely supported along its entire length and there is no weight on her stomach. As one woman reported, "I loved watching my husband's face from this position—I was so relaxed when he was inside of me, and I just got into the pleasure without any awareness of anything else." Another woman said, "I have always had to be careful about my back, and after delivering Gaylene, I found I needed a really supportive position without Gary's weight on me. The Kneeling at the Altar, as we call it, has become our best position."

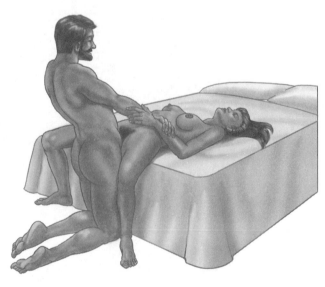

Fig. 36

G Spot Stimulation

Most couples find there are physical changes in the woman's genitals that have to be taken into account after a vaginal delivery, which we described in Chapter Eleven. The introitus, the opening into the vagina, may feel more open, or if there was an episiotomy, tighter, due to the healing, shrinking scar tissue. There is good news, however, for those women who enjoy G spot stimulation: a vaginal delivery actually makes that type of pleasuring more intense and easier once you've delivered this way.

During a private seminar, I was relating the research information of Dr. Lasse Hessel, who showed the most intense vaginal canal stimulation areas of couples in various positions using ultrasound photography. With a vaginal delivery, the interior of the canal becomes more elastic. As a result, during penetration, especially rear-entry doggie-style penetration, the head of the man's glans will be stroking directly over the G spot area. I remember well one woman in a private seminar who did not speak English very well trying to describe her favorite position to her friend. Finally she got down on all fours, lowered her shoulders, and said, "Theese way, theese way." She also pointed out that after her baby was born the sensation was even better—and now she knew why.

The Lift and Separate Cunnilingus Technique

A mother of three shared with me how she hadn't had an orgasm in almost a year when previously she'd had them easily, especially when her husband gave her oral sex. She discovered that a particular technique worked very well for her. As she related to me, "It was like he lifted everything up with his fingers and whamo—I came fast and furious, just like before. I hadn't realized how much things had shifted down there." So she and her husband practice the "lift and separate" technique.

This technique is described by men in the know as the best way to gain access to a woman's most sensitive parts. The man is lying between the lady's legs or next to her side. First he uses the clean fingers of one hand to gently spread open the outer and inner labia (lips). He then uses both hands to lift and/or push up the fleshy mons pubis to expose the ultrasensitive clitoral glans.

Stay Neat and Tidy Down There

One woman described the change in her genitals in this way: "After three children, it has become more important to keep everything neat and tidy. I always trim my pubic hair and present things in terrific lingerie."

Tantric Techniques

Couples who have just birthed a child often assume the philosophy of tantric sex without realizing they are doing so. The slow, connecting deep-breathing positions favored by tantric sex practitioners take on a new meaning after a baby when couples often choose slower more emotionally filled sex as they reenter the physical arena of expressing their love for one another. This is intimacy that is more about who they are for one another than just what their bodies need or are. Also at a time when couples are often not having as much sex as they did before, the power of tantric sexuality can have them connect more deeply and more intensely.

Before you say to yourself, "Oh, please," let me remind you that breathing and being centered emotionally with your partner are the tenets of any great intimacy. And never overlook that orgasms are powered by blood and oxygen, both of which are increased with yogic breathing practices.

Tantric sex is just that: the study of the ability to breathe in conjunction with your lover, expanding your breath and connection to other levels of awareness and sensation. Who wouldn't want a partner who is focused on the two of you and being mindful of whatever he needs to do to do so? According to Margot Anand, a tantric sex expert and the author of *The Art of Sexual Ecstasy*, there are three keys to orgasmic power: 1) breathing with attention; 2) movement with feeling; 3) voice with expression. "Proper breathing relaxes and energizes the body, clarifies and focuses the mind, and opens us up to new depths of sensual/emotional feeling, which can then be expressed and enhanced through vocal expression. When we are so 'attuned,' our speech becomes Eros, part of the play of our lovemaking."

Here are a few positions to consider:

YAB YUM

In figure 37 the classic Yab Yum allows the couple to be as close as possible yet still free to move. Their chakras, the energy points along the body that tantric practitioners are aware of, are at the same levels thanks to the pillow under the lady's derriere. This position puts the woman in charge of motion for, as you all know, the partner on top controls the motion. This allows her to maintain full penetration that

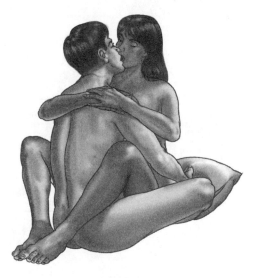

Fig. 37

she is comfortable with and to control the depth of penetration she prefers while being fully supported by pillows and his encircling arms.

Here, depending on closeness, either partner can add manual stimulation to their play. As one woman described, "I love getting into the Yab Yum position and leaning my body back so that I can watch my husband entering me. This position, hands down, is one of my biggest turn-ons. I get even hotter when I am the one controlling the show. When I am sitting on top of him, I can see his penis arching into me, and then he uses his hand to do me—ooohh, baby, doesn't get any better!!"

Position 38 is for those couples who still have free range of their home. As new parents many couples want to reaffirm that they still have the spontaneous attitude "there isn't a surface in our house we won't play on." Any new location outside the bedroom can be your playground. Figure 38 shows a couple enjoying their low coffee table for more than hors d'oeuvres. Best to use a towel on a flat surface so her back doesn't get cold. Should she prefer, she can move her heels to his shoulders to vary sensation or her knees farther apart for manual stimulation.

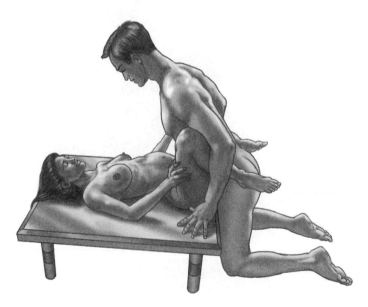

Fig. 38

I have gathered a few more subtle tantric techniques suggested by Charles and Caroline Muir in their inspired *Tantra: The Art of Conscious Loving.*

DELIGHTING THE ONE WHO KNEELS ABOVE
(AKA SOMF—SIT ON MY FACE, POSITION 32. SEE PAGE 151)

This is a form of oral sex in which the woman kneels above her man's mouth. The man is passive and receives the woman onto his mouth. The woman then uses "1001 gentle or subtle pelvic movements to find her own pleasure." You may not need all 1001.

THE KISS OF THE LOWER LIP

Should kissing be your preferred method of opening up your sexual world, try the kiss of the lower lip. Start kissing your lover, and then gently pull his lower lip into your mouth. With the tip of your tongue stroke a quarter-inch line along the sexual meridian line, which runs from the exterior outer edge of the lower lip to where the lip attaches to the chin.

Dr. Phil McGraw dedicated his bestselling book *Relationship Rescue* to his wife. His very poignant and honest comment was this: "This book is dedicated with love and gratitude to my wife, Robin, who never stopped being a wife even though she became a mother." As you come to the end of this book, I would like you to ponder this dedication. If it rings true to you, then you have transformed yourself into a Hot Mama.

A Final Note

THIS BOOK IS FOR ALL pregnant women and new mothers. It was written because many women asked me what they needed to know to make sure their sex lives weren't derailed during pregnancy or by having children. They knew that their bodies and their lives would be altered—a fact of life—yet they wanted to know exactly what they could do to better prepare themselves and their relationships. They knew as parents they were entering this entity called family for the long haul, and approaching it as if it were a marathon. And as with a marathon, these women knew you must train: collect information about how to better your experience, and prepare for ill weather and rocky terrain.

So whether you are pregnant, a new mother, or a new father, this book contains the material you can use to ensure that the intimacy that created your child is maintained throughout your marathon—your pregnancy and long after. Motherhood is a one-way street, and you have assumed this role for the rest of your life, so relish it, cherish it, and most of all make it work for you and your partner. Know that eventually your life will assume an even keel and your sex life will do the same. Will they be changed? Yes. Do you have to have a commitment and a willingness to flow with the changes? Yes. Is it worth it? Yes. Change is inherent in being alive, and life is about how we embrace change.

No one can describe the challenge that comes with pregnancy and parenthood better than those who have been through it. Consider what this New York father of two, whose wife works, said: "Sometimes my wife and I are so tired that sex is the last thing on our minds. Then we realize how much we miss that feeling of being connected with each other, and how much we need it while we are building our lives, our family, and our futures together. It's a huge part of us." This desire and need for connection—at all levels—was echoed by many women and men with whom I spoke.

I also feel strongly that any mother should be acknowledged for the huge amount of work creating and taking care of children can be. As a mother of three said, "If women actually knew how much work being a mother was going to be, I think more of them would have thought twice about doing it. Yet there is nothing, absolutely nothing that has given my life more richness or fulfillment." So there's the rub. There is probably never going to be another event that will as dramatically change every part of your life—especially your intimate life—as a pregnancy.

After listening to thousands of expectant and new parents, I have deduced the "magic formula" for not having your relationship lose its luster and intimacy once you become a parent: bless yourselves and your relationship with the *attitude and intention* of keeping your sex life healthy. Simple words, I know, yet I also know the simplest information is often the most powerful. In speaking to couples worldwide, I am constantly reminded of what keeps Hot Mamas hot whether their children are three months old or thirteen years old. . . . It is in the heartbeat of that attitude and their behavior.

I truly hope you learn from the Hot Mamas you encountered in this book, who have shared their experiences of dealing with the huge life and relationship transitions that occur when you become a mother, a parent. And I wish you all the best as you enter the world of parenthood—be it for the first or the ninth time. I know from listening to those who have gone before you that these insights and experiences have the power to take your relationship to the next level. So just as your intimate relationship adapted and adjusted to all of pregnancy's four trimesters, know that it will continue to change throughout your life. Keep the spirit of being a Hot Mama alive, and you, your relationship, and your children will thrive.

Enjoy.

Lou Paget

Bibliography

American Academy of Pediatrics, American College of Obstetricians and Gynecologists. *Guidelines for Perinatal Care*, 5th ed. Elk Grove Village, IL, and Washington, DC: ACOG/AAP, 2002.

American College of Obstetricians and Gynecologists. *Planning Your Pregnancy and Birth*, 3rd ed. Washington, DC: ACOG, 2000.

Anand, Margo. *The Art of Sexual Ecstasy: The Path of Sacred Sexuality for Western Lovers*. Los Angeles: Jeremy P. Tarcher, Inc., 1989.

Bischof, Guscetti, and Karoline Susanne, M.D., Ph.D. "Women's Sexuality After Childbirth." Ph. D. diss., presented to the Institute for Advanced Study of Human Sexuality, San Francisco, in partial fulfillment of the requirements for the degree of doctor of philosophy, 2004.

Black, Jules, M.D. *Body Talk: An A–Z Guide to Women's Health*. Sydney, Australia: Angus & Robertson Publishers, 1988.

———. (1990) "Oxytocin: The 'Love Hormone.'" Proceedings, 6th Advanced Course, Royal Australian College of Obstetricians & Gynæcologists, Adelaide, South Australia, May 13–15, 1990.

Boland, Katie. *I Got Pregnant, You Can Too! How Healing Yourself Physically, Mentally and Spiritually Leads to Fertility*. Grass Valley, CA: Underwood Books, 1998.

Brazelton, T. Berry, M.D., and Sparrow, Joshua D., M.D. *Sleep: The Brazelton Way*. Cambridge, MA: Perseus, 2003.

Brott, Armin A., and Ash, Jennifer. *The Expectant Father: Facts, Tips, and Advice for Dads-to-Be*, 2nd ed. New York: Abbeville Press, 2001.

Chang, Stephen T. *The Tao of Sexology: The Book of Infinite Wisdom*. Reno, NV: Tao Publishing, 1986.

Cunningham, F. Gary et al. *Williams Obstetrics*, 21st ed. New York: McGraw-Hill, 2001.

Curtis, Glade B., M.D., OB/GYN, and Schuler, Judith, M.S. *Your Pregnancy for the Father-to-Be: Everything Dads Need to Know About Pregnancy, Childbirth, and Getting Ready for a New Baby.* Cambridge, MA: Perseus, 2003.

Curtis, Glade B., M.D., FACOG. *Your Pregnancy Week by Week.* Tucson, AZ: Fisher Books, 1994.

Davis Raskin, Valerie, M.D. *Great Sex for Moms: Ten Steps to Nurturing Passion While Raising* Kids. New York: Simon & Schuster, 2002.

Douglas, Ann. *The Mother of All Pregnancy Books: The Ultimate Guide to Conception, Birth, and Everything in Between.* New York: Hungry Minds, 2002.

Eiger, Marvin S. and Olds, Sally Wendkos. *The Complete Book of Breastfeeding: The Classic Guide for Every Nursing Mother.* New York: Bantam, 1999.

Eisenberg, Arlene, Murkoff, Heidi E., and Hathaway, Sandee E., B.S.N. *What to Expect When You're Expecting, 2nd Edition.* New York: Workman, 1996.

Fisher, Helen. *The First Sex: The Natural Talents of Women and How They Are Changing the World.* New York: Random House, 1999.

Ganem, Marc B., M.D. *La Sexualité du couple pendant la grossesse: guide pratique.* Paris, France: Filipacchi, 1992.

Gaskin, Ina May. *Ina May's Guide to Childbirth.* New York: Bantam, 2003.

Gliksman, Michele Isaacs, M.D., and DiGeronimo, Theresa Foy. *The Complete Idiot's Guide to Pregnancy and Childbirth.* Indianapolis: Alpha Books, 1999.

Gurmukh. *Bountiful, Beautiful, Blissful: Experience the Natural Power of Pregnancy and Birth with Kundalini Yoga and Meditation.* New York: St. Martin's Press, 2003.

Hale, Thomas W., Ph.D. *Medications and Mother's Milk*, 11th ed. Amarillo, TX: Pharmasoft Publishing, 2002.

Hoge, Hilary, M.D. *Women's Stories of Divorce at Childbirth: When the Baby Rocks the Cradle.* New York: The Haworth Clinical Practice Press, Inc., 2002.

Lernere, Henry M., M.D., OB/GYN. *Miscarriage: A Doctor's Guide to the Facts.* Cambridge, MA: Perseus, 2003.

Manning, John T. *Digit Ratio: A Pointer to Fertility, Behavior, and Health.* New Brunswick, NJ: Rutgers University Press, 2002.

Margot, Sandra, C.C.S., A.C.S. *The Pregnant Couple's Guide to Sex, Romance and Intimacy.* New York: Kensington Publishing Corp., 2002.

McGraw, Phillip C., Ph.D. *Relationship Rescue: A Seven-Step Strategy for Reconnecting with Your Partner.* New York: Hyperion, 2000.

Mohr, Ralf. *Pregnant: Nudes by Ralf Mohr.* Munich, Germany: Edition Reuss, 1998.

Nathanielsz, Peter, M.D., Ph.D., with Christopher Vaughan. *The Prenatal Prescription*. New York: Quill, 2002.

Pepper, Rachel. *The Ultimate Guide to Pregnancy for Lesbians: Tips and Techniques from Conception Through Birth*. San Francisco: Cleis Press, 1999.

Richmond, Cynthia. *Dream Power: How to Use Your Night Dreams to Change Your Life*. New York: Fireside, 2000.

Salmansohn, Karen. *Hot Mama: How to Have a Babe and Be a Babe*. San Francisco: Chronicle Books, 2003.

Schulz, Mona Lisa, M.D., Ph.D. *Awakening Intuition: Using Your Mind-Body Network for Insight and Healing*. New York: Three Rivers Press, 1998.

Smith, Caroline, Ph.D., M.S., et al. "A Randomized Controlled Trial of Ginger to Treat Nausea and Vomiting in Pregnancy." *The American College of Obstetricians and Gynecologists* (103) (2004): pp. 639–645.

Stewart, Elizabeth G., and Spencer, Paula. *The V Book: A Doctor's Guide to Complete Vulvovaginal Health*. New York: Bantam Books, 2002.

Stone, Joanne, M.D., Eddleman, Keith, M.D., and Murray, Mary. *Pregnancy for Dummies*. New York: Hungry Minds, 1999.

Stoppard, Miriam, M.D. *Conception, Pregnancy & Birth: The Childbirth Bible for Today's Parents*. New York: Dorling Kindersley Publishing, Inc., 2000.

Venning, Rachel, and Cavanah, Claire. *Sex Toys 101: A Playfully Uninhibited Guide*. New York: Fireside, 2003.

Von Sydow, Kirsten, Ph.D. "Sexuality During Pregnancy and After Childbirth: A Metacontent Analysis of 59 Studies." *Journal of Psychosomatic Research* (47, no. 1) (1999): 27–49.

Whipple, Beverly, Ph.D. et al. "Inverse Relationship Between Intensity of Vaginal Self-stimulation-Produced Analgesia and Level of Chronic Intake of a Dietary Source of Capsaicin." *Physiology & Behavior* (46) (1989): 247–252.

Index